45⁰⁰

WHO CARES?

Who Cares?

THEORY, RESEARCH, AND EDUCATIONAL IMPLICATIONS OF THE ETHIC OF CARE

EDITED BY

Mary M. Brabeck

PRAEGER

New York
Westport, Connecticut
London

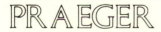

Copyright Acknowledgments

Bill Puka's essay, "The Liberation of Caring: A Different Voice for Gilligan's 'Different Voice'" is reprinted here by permission from *Hypatia*.

Earlier versions of the following appeared in *The Journal of Moral Education* 16 (3), 1987: A version of "Ways of Knowing, Learning and Making Moral Choices" by Nona Lyons; parts of "The Just Community Educational Program: The Development of Moral Role-Taking as the Expression of Justice and Care" by Ann Higgins appeared as "A Feminist Perspective on Moral Education"; "Transforming Moral Education" by Jane Roland Martin appeared under the same title; parts of "Ethical Sensitivity and Moral Reasoning among Men and Women in the Professions" by Muriel Bebeau and Mary Brabeck appeared in "Integrating Care and Justice Issues in Professional Moral Education: A Gender Perspective"; and a version of "Educating Good People" by Nel Noddings, appeared as "Do We Really Want to Produce Good People?" These sections are reprinted by permission of NFER-NELSON, Windsor, U.K.

Library of Congress Cataloging-in-Publication Data

Who cares? : theory, research, and educational implications of the
  ethic of care / edited by Mary M. Brabeck.
     p.   cm.
   Bibliography: p.
   Includes index.
   ISBN 0–275–93253–2 (alk. paper)
    1. Women—Psychology. 2. Caring. 3. Femininity (Psychology)
4. Feminism.   I. Brabeck, Mary M.
HQ1206.W64   1989   89–3911

Library of Congress Catalog Card Number: 89-3911
ISBN: 0-275-93253-2

First published in 1989

Praeger Publishers, One Madison Avenue, New York, NY 10010
A division of Greenwood Press, Inc.

Printed in the United States of America

∞

The paper used in this book complies with the Permanent Paper Standard issued by the National Information Standards Organization (Z39.48–1984).

10 9 8 7 6 5 4 3 2 1

To Michael, David, and Kalina, who really do care.

Contents

Acknowledgments

I am grateful to the contributors of this volume who put up with my many phone calls, letters, and revised plans, and who met my deadlines. I thank Lisa Kuhmerker for prompting me to begin this project, my family for helping me persist, and Karen Weisgerber and Alison Bricken for helping me finish. Boston College provided a faculty research grant that enabled me to circulate draft copies among the participants in the project.

Introduction: Who Cares?

Mary Brabeck

Two major shifts that have occurred in contemporary thinking about the human condition are reflected in this volume. The first shift arises from critiques of descriptions of human nature as autonomous, independent, individualistic, and rational and of the moral ideal as principled, objective, rationally apprehended, and universal. Contemporary scholars are claiming that the self does not exist apart from relationships, that one is interconnected with others in essential ways, and that the moral ideal includes responsibility toward others, connection, and compassion.

The second shift in contemporary thinking involves a change in feminist theories. Over the past two decades, feminist theorists have increasingly moved away from attempts to attain equality by calling attention to similarities between males and females, toward a celebration of gender differences. These two events, the redefinition of human nature and the moral ideal, and the change in the attitudes about gender differences are joined in the discussions about "who cares" offered in this book.

In 1971 Elizabeth Janeway presaged the critique of the autonomous, separate individual. Comparing the decade of the 1960s to that of the 1970s Janeway wrote, "Where we once boasted that we are free, we are now more inclined to fear we are alienated" (Janeway 1971, p. 75). Robert Bellah and his colleagues (Bellah et al. 1985) have sounded the alarm on the limits of American individualism revealed in their interviews with people across the United States. The enormous popularity of this book reflects an unease with and distrust of the individualistic ideal. This longing for a sense of community, a joining with others, is also reflected in the 1988 United States presidential election slogans which focused on the family unit and called for a "kinder, gentler" nation.

The proclivity of contemporary Western culture to embrace individual autonomy and personal freedom has led us to advocate, out of Hobbesian concerns, that human rights be protected, civil rights be assured, and equal rights be attained. However, recently we have come to see the limits of a moral view that is based entirely on concerns about individual rights and which ignores responsibility to and inclusion of others (Bellah et al. 1985; Cancian 1987).

At the same time that social critics have described the limitations of our current moral ideal, there has been a change in feminist theorists' attitudes about difference, particularly differences in moral vision and sensitivity.

The tendency in Western culture to dichotomize, reason–emotion, fact–value, good–evil, culture–nature, masculine–feminine, etc., assumes a hierarchy of opposites in which the first attribute is valued over the second. In contemporary society this tendency to dichotomize has been extended to individualism–community, autonomy–relatedness, competition–coopera- tion, rights–responsibilities. These, too, have been related to gender, and the tasks, attributes, and roles assigned to men have been valued over those assigned to women. To prevent researchers from drawing conclusions that devalue women or support maintaining her inferior status, feminist researchers have tried in the past to refute claims of differences between men and women. They have pointed out that there are very few reliably found gender differences (e.g. Maccoby and Jacklin 1974) and that where differences between males and females have been demonstrated the actual magnitude of statistical difference is very small (e.g., Hyde and Linn 1986). They have drawn attention to the value-biased interpretation of studies that have found gender differences and have defined the ideal person as an- drogynous (e.g. Bem 1974; Heilbrun 1973; Spence and Helmreich 1978). Androgyny theories, buttressed by reports such as Maccoby and Jacklin's (1974), suggested that women could be autonomous, competitive, analytic, dominant, and aggressive as males.

However, it has become evident that in the androgynous view, the feminine qualities of sensitivity, and of being affectionate, cheerful, childlike, gentle, compassionate, and gullible (Bem 1974), are not as valued as the masculine qualities (Eisenstein 1983). Furthermore, androgyny theories maintain the androcentric view of the superior qualities of males by suggesting that male qualities should simply be mapped onto females to achieve a whole person. Recently theorists have argued that women ought not rush to be born again in the masculine norm, when that norm is fun- damentally flawed (Miller 1984). Joining the critics of individualism and autonomy as hallmarks of the human person, they have pointed out the in- adequacy of the masculine, autonomous, competitive, and hierarchical model. They have called, instead, for new, feminist models that affirm the alternative feminine values and virtues (Gilligan 1982; Miller 1976; Ruddick 1980).

This shift away from refuting gender differences and toward celebrating differences has its foundation in what has been called a woman-centered analysis. As outlined by the historian Gerda Lerner (1979), and applied in the analysis of the sociologist Nancy Chodorow (1978) and the psychologist Jean Baker Miller (1976), among others, a women-centered analysis "located specific virtues in the historical and psychological experience of women. Instead of seeking to minimize the polarization between masculine and feminine," a woman-centered analysis "sought to isolate and to define those aspects of female experience that were potential sources of strength and power for women" (Eisenstein 1983, p. xii).

The work of the architects of the ethic of care (Gilligan 1982; Martin 1985; Noddings 1984) falls into this post-androgyny period of feminist theory. During the decade of the 1980s they and other theorists identified an alternative to the celebration of the autonomous individual. Feminist scholars have turned to the experience of women, who traditionally have been associated with care-giving and relationship building in family and community, to describe an ethic directed toward reducing alienation. From what Carol Gilligan (1982) called "a different voice," an ethic of care emerged as the central concern guiding and fostering development and maintenance of relationships. Gilligan contrasted the ethic of care with the ethic of justice, which she labeled a masculine norm, described and researched by Kohlberg and colleagues (Kohlberg 1969; Kohlberg, Levine and Hewer 1983). Through interviews about their personally experienced moral dilemmas, as well as their informal theories of morality, Gilligan found evidence that care was more likely to be found among girls and women than among boys and men.

Nel Noddings (1984) identified caring as the moral virtue necessary for reducing alienation and guiding moral action. The motivation toward ethical caring, she claimed, arises out of natural caring, love, out of a longing to be in caring, committed relationships. She extended her analysis from the receptivity and responsivity characteristic of the caring mother-child relationship, to the teacher-student relationship and examined the implications for curriculum changes that follow from the ethic of caring.

Jane Roland Martin (1985) analyzed recommendations for women's education, from the writings of Plato, Rousseau, Wolstonecraft, Beecher, and Gilman. She contrasted the individualistic, rational ideal that emerges from philosophical discussions of education for citizenship, with the relational, caring ideal that emerges from philosophical discussion of the education of women. Arguing for a "gender sensitive" approach to education, she asserted that educational endeavors must be deliberately attentive to the ways in which gender views have affected our ideal of the educated person. Only then, she suggests, will generative love be valued and incorporated in ways that transform our educational structures.

The ethic of care has received a great deal of attention in both popular and professional arenas. This book brings together the work of scholars who have been critiquing and extending the ethic of care and its claims to being gender related. Contributors to this volume assume readers have some familiarity with these recent feminist theories of care. Summary and discussion of Carol Gilligan's ethic of care appear in chapters by Bill Puka, Nona Lyons, and Muriel Bebeau and myself. Summaries of Nel Noddings's theory of caring appear in both her own and in Barbara Houston's chapters. Summaries of Jane Roland Martin's work on the ideal that emerges from writings about the education of women likewise appear in her own and in Nel Noddings's chapters.

These chapters also extend the work of the theorists who have described the ethic of care. In Part I of this book the writers define and redefine the nature of care, examine its philosophical base, and illuminate its political ramifications. In Part II the empirical validity of claims about the relationship between care and gender is scrutinized, the relationship between moral vision, epistemology, and views of the self are examined, psychological studies of constructs related to the ethic of care are summarized, and the socialization factors that affect the development of caring responses and the caring self are discussed. In Part III, the ethic of care is examined in current and proposed educational models, and the educational transformations necessary to develop caring persons are suggested. However, such divisions are somewhat artificial; many writers in this collection combine philosophical analysis, empirical observations, and educational recommendations.

There is controversy in the works presented here. Authors were sent early drafts of papers. Some contributors address issues raised in this volume with which they disagree; some extend and support the arguments of other authors; all address the question "who cares?" from the different perspectives of their academic disciplines: philosophy, psychology, theology, and education.

Mary Ellen Waithe begins our discussion of the ethic of care by placing the ethic within an historical context of the writings of early women philosophers. She presents three versions of moral theory that are extant in the work of women philosophers as early as circa 350 B.C. Tracing the evolution of their theories through two milennia, she reveals a gradual evolution toward a gender undifferentiated view of morality. These early philosophical writings, she argues, suggest the possibility of synthesizing the virtues of justice and care within an undifferentiated moral philosophy.

Waithe's chapter reminds us that the ethic of care has a philosophical history. She finds in the work of ancient women philosophers many of the issues taken up by contributors to this volume. Thus, she sets the stage for the discussions in the chapters that follow. These include the nature of care, the gender relatedness of care, the political and psychological price of attributing care to women, the socialization experiences that shape and develop the caring response and the caring self, the relationship between

care and rationality and between care and justice, and the distinction between a theory of care based on social morality (the norms of society) and
theoretical morality (moral philosophy).

Bill Puka takes up many of these issues in Chapter 2 in his examination of
the levels of care in Carol Gilligan's theory. Citing evidence from her empirical work, he suggests that Gilligan's ethic of care may not be the broad
moral orientation she claims it to be. Rather, he argues, in a patriarchal
society care may be a strategy for coping with sexism. Puka's "care as
liberation" hypothesis suggests that the caring response may be understood
not as sequential, holistic, moral development, but as skills or ideologies
that assume different forms (Gilligan's levels of care). The "care as liberation" hypothesis suggests that these skills or ideologies result from sexist
socialization of women into a service orientation.

In the third chapter Toinette Eugene traces the subjugation and exploitation of black women to examine the liberational ethic of care that has been
forged out of their experience. Her argument, grounded in the biblical and
religious context of the African-American experience, celebrates the black
women who have assumed the role of servant–leader in their communities.
The moral vision that arises from their particular cultural context includes
connection and care, as well as the just struggle for liberation.

Charlene Haddock Seigfried provides a philosophical basis for contextual
theories of morality in Chapter 4. Equating claims to universality, neutrality, and objectivity with the drive for dominance, she argues that any moral
theory must be judged by the consequences, the outcomes, that follow from
one's moral view. Thus, she focuses attention on the conditions that bring
about different ethical responses and argues that attending sympathetically
and with feeling, to the particular concerns and needs of others, is prerequisite for justice and for a morality of care.

Barbara Houston, in Chapter 5, asks whether an ethic of caring can avoid
self-sacrifice. She probes the issue of the cost of women's caring, the role of
caring in maintaining women's powerlessness and oppression. She argues
that women's caring has been invisible and devalued and she attributes
women's struggles for self-assertion and stronger self-image with moral
significance. While she asserts that the ethic of care ought to be retained,
Houston's analysis demonstrates that the claims that care is gender related
are problematic from both philosophical and political perspectives.

In Chapter 6 Nona Lyons extends the discussion of care as moral vision
to include the connected self. She draws from her work with Carol Gilligan
in researching the ethic of care, and from her recent investigation of adolescent girls' ways of knowing. Lyons presented a model in which the learners'
interests and goals and their approaches to knowing are related to their conceptions of self and morality. While she maintains that ways of knowing
and moral orientation are gender related, she demonstrates the diversity
among adolescent women in their focus on moral and epistemological

issues. Her work suggests that when developmental models are made available to teachers, teaching strategies may better match the students' approaches to learning.

In Chapter 7, Nancy Eisenberg, Richard Fabes, and Cindy Shea summarize the literature related to claims that girls and women are more "other-oriented" and sympathetic to the plight of others. They review the social-cognitive psychological literature on gender differences in emotional responsivity, empathy, and prosocial moral reasoning. They present evidence that suggests that differential socialization patterns result in small but observed gender differences in psychological constructs related to the ethic of care.

After reviewing the burgeoning literature on gender differences in justice and care moral orientations, Muriel Bebeau and I suggest in the eighth chapter that educators and researchers need to carefully define the component of morality being considered. We propose that the ethic of care be conceptualized as one component of morality, ethical sensitivity, rather than as a comprehensive developmental theory of moral reasoning, or alternative to Kohlberg's stage theory. We present empirical evidence that males and females at the same educational level differ in ethical sensitivity but not in recognition of issues of care and justice, nor in principled moral reasoning.

In Chapter 9 M. Brinton Lykes returns to the issues of the impact of oppression and powerlessness on the development of the ethic of care. Her analysis leads her to construct care as "social individuality." Lykes locates this ethic primarily among women working at lower paying jobs who have been actively engaged in resistance to or struggle against oppressive systems. Lykes demonstrates through studies of black mothers, her own previous research, and recent interviews with Guatemalan women in exile, that the collective experience and the economic, historical, and political reality of that experience, is critical in the development of one's sense of self and moral vision.

When feminine qualities such as care, sensitivity, and empathy are included in descriptions of the educational ideal, educational structures may be radically transformed. In Chapter 10, Jane Roland Martin traces the cultural ideal of the educated person through the works of Plato and Rousseau to examine its genderized roots. While Barbara Houston (Chapter 5) worries that girls and women may care too much, Martin worries that boys and men may care too little. She calls upon educators to incorporate the reproductive processes typically assigned to females, with the productive processes typically assigned to males, and argues that a feminist perspective on moral education mandates a redefinition not only of our cultural ideal but of education itself.

Ann Higgins has worked extensively in Kohlbergian moral development programs, most recently in the Bronx schools system, using a just community approach. Drawing from this work, she argues in Chapter 11 that care can be expressed only in the context of justice. Thus, she rejects relativistic values in favor of the principles of equality and equity, defining concepts of liberal feminism. She reports on an ongoing program in a large inner city school system in the Bronx. She uses excerpts from interviews with students in the program to describe how the just community program uses moral role taking to foster development of care through the development of justice.

In the final chapter of this book, Nel Noddings describes the masculinist warrior model and the feminine-feminist maternal model and their views of good and evil. She addresses the disturbing question: Do we really want to educate good people? Her analysis demonstrates that educators are yet a long way from achieving the moral ideal of caring suggested by a feminine-feminist perspective. She then moves beyond critique to suggest the educational content and methods that hold potential for movement toward the moral ideal.

The contributors to this volume articulate a moral view that historically has been associated with women and has been called the feminine virtues: care, concern, and connection (Martin 1985). The work presented here may be seen as marking a transition via a woman-centered analysis to a reformulated theory of androgyny in which these values are normative. In a reversal of earlier theories of androgyny, in which the masculine was mapped onto the female, this view joins what has been called the feminine virtues with what has been called the masculine virtues in a vision of a mature moral person. The moral ideal that follows reflects reasoned, deliberate judgments that ensure justice be accorded each individual while maintaining a deep concern for the well-being of all people. This moral ideal is directed toward transcendence of masculine and feminine aims and virtues and calls upon all to care.

REFERENCES

Bellah, R., Madsen, R., Sullivan, W., Swidler, A., and Tipton, S. (1985). *Habits of the heart: Individualism and commitment in American life*. New York: Harper & Row.

Bem, S. (1974). The measurement of psychological androgyny. *Journal of Consulting and Clinical Psychology* 42: 155–162.

Cancian, F. (1987). *Love in America: Gender and self-development*. Cambridge: Cambridge University Press.

Chodorow, N. (1978). *The reproduction of mothering: Psychoanalysis and the sociology of gender*. Berkeley: University of California Press.

Eisenstein, H. (1983). *Contemporary feminist thought*. Boston: G. K. Hall & Co.

Gilligan, C. (1982). *In a different voice: Psychological theory and women's development*. Cambridge, MA: Harvard University Press.

Heilbrun, C. (1973). *Toward a recognition of androgyny*. New York: Harper & Row.

Hyde, J. S., and Linn, M. C., eds. (1986). *The psychology of gender: Advances through meta-analysis*. Baltimore: Johns Hopkins University Press.

Janeway, E. (1971). *Man's world, woman's place: A study in social mythology*. New York: Dell Publishing Co.

Kohlberg, L. (1969). Stage and sequence: The cognitive-developmental approach to socialization. In *Handbook of socialization theory and research*, ed. D. A. Goslin. Chicago: Rand McNally.

Kohlberg, L., Levine, C., and Hewer, A. (1983). *Moral stages: A current formulation and a response to critics*. Basel: S. Karger.

Lerner, G. (1979). *The majority finds its past: Placing women in history*. New York: Oxford University Press.

Maccoby, E. E., and Jacklin, C. N. (1974). *The psychology of sex differences*. Stanford, CA: Stanford University Press.

Martin, J. R. (1985). *Reclaiming a conversation*. New Haven: Yale University Press.

Miller, J. B. (1984. *The development of women's sense of self*. (Working Papers in Progress, No. 84–01). Wellesley, MA: Wellesley College, The Stone Center.

———. (1976). *Toward a new psychology of women*. Boston: Beacon Press.

Noddings, N. (1984). *Caring: a feminine approach to ethics and moral education*. Berkeley, CA: University of California Press.

Ruddick, S. (1980). Maternal thinking. *Feminist Studies* 5 (2): 342–367.

Spence, J. T., and Helmreich, R. L. (1978). *Masculinity and femininity: The psychological dimensions, correlates and antecedents*. Austin, TX: University of Texas Press.

Part I

DEFINING AND REDEFINING
THE ETHIC OF CARE

Twenty-three Hundred Years of Women Philosophers: Toward a Gender Undifferentiated Moral Theory

Mary Ellen Waithe

Carol Gilligan's (1982) argument as presented in *In A Different Voice* begins by responding to aspects of Kohlberg's moral development theory, and continues in her recent work "Moral Orientation and Moral Development" (Gilligan 1987), where she responds to "moral theory" in general. In her published works Gilligan does not explicitly link her argument to earlier philosophical arguments, nor does she place her view in a larger, historical context. As Annette Baier (1987) notes, Gilligan's response *appears* to be a response to the same historical tradition within which Kohlberg's theory has developed: the "justice tradition" represented by the moral philosophies of John Rawls (twentieth century), Immanuel Kant (nineteenth century) and John Locke (seventeenth century). And although these writers borrowed some elements from the tradition of Plato (fifth to fourth centuries *B.C.*), the "justice tradition" is only 300 years old. Gilligan's argument is directed against this relatively recent tradition. Gilligan's focus on that particular philosophic tradition may convey the impression that moral philosophy per se is exclusively justice-oriented. As Baier notes, there is another tradition in moral theory, the "virtue tradition." Although Hume (1711–1776) is the foremost modern proponent of the virtue tradition, it is one which extends as far back as Aristotle.

Gilligan's most recent work offers a distinction " . . . between care as understood or construed within a justice framework and care as a framework or a perspective on moral decision" (Gilligan 1987, p. 24). In the framework of the justice tradition, care is represented as the mercy which tempers justice, or, the decision to care is represented as a decision to "modulate" justice by introducing other considerations. Gilligan notes that although the care framework is less fleshed out than the justice framework, it is grounded in assumptions about the mutual interdependence of persons, in responsiveness rather than in reciprocity, in relationships rather than in selves.

The works of many women philosophers discussed in this chapter are difficult to classify as belonging either to the justice or virtue traditions, although those works clearly present a care perspective. When the care framework becomes more fully fleshed out, it may turn out to be another theory within the "virtue" tradition. This in turn leads me to question whether Gilligan's distinction between "care" and "justice" overlooks some fundamental synthesis of the two perspectives under which they ought to be mutually reducible to a perspective of gender undifferentiated human morality.

Is there one morality, and does it include care and justice? *Is* morality gender related? Gilligan's (and by extension, others, including Noddings [1984], Martin [1985], and Ruddick [1984]) identification of women with a care-oriented philosophical construct appears new when considered against the background of recent moral philosophy. In this chapter I present an historical perspective which includes the views of women philosophers of the past two milennia. When women philosophers' views are examined, we see a gradual evolution toward a gender undifferentiated view of morality, a view in which one can recognize elements of both the justice and virtue traditions. Three versions of the gender undifferentiated view emerge in the writings of women philosophers.

The earliest version of the gender undifferentiated view holds that 'care' and 'justice' are mutually dependent constructs at the level of theory even if, at the level of social practice, acts of 'caring' are attributed to women, and acts of 'justice' are attributed to men. According to this view, at the level of moral theory, action cannot be morally right unless it is both caring and just. Consequently, it would make no sense to speak of either gender's capacity for morally right action exclusively in terms of that gender's social role which may impose special responsibilities for care or for justice. A second, and more complexly argued version holds that men and women are both capable of morality. A consequence of this version of the gender undifferentiated view is that women are morally entitled to equal social rights because they are men's moral equals. A third version of the gender undifferentiated view holds that even if care and justice are independent moral constructs, and even if there are gender differences in the capacity for care or for justice, those differences are not significant enough to be morally relevant. In this chapter, I shall examine the history of the slow evolution of a gender undifferentiated view of women's capacity for morality within each of these three traditions.

ONE MORALITY—CARE AND JUSTICE

The earliest documented moral theory (from circa sixth century *B.C.)* considered the soul to be the locus of moral capacity. From at least the time of Pythagoras' doctrine of reincarnation, the soul of a woman was considered to be halfway between that of an animal and that of a man. Only the souls of virtuous men were considered to be capable of achieving immortality. Although this is an oversimplified account of a philosophy that dominated moral theory in the ancient world until the early centuries after Christ, even the most egalitarian moral philosophers like Plato (fourth century *B.C.*), claimed that women had souls but were capable only of inferior virtue (Plato, *Timeaus*, 42c.).[1] There have always been theories of moral philosophy which have considered both virtue and justice to be necessary features of morally right action. This view has explicitly characterized almost all of moral theory.[2]

Historically, one of the most important moral principles has been the principle of care and concern for others. Moral philosophy in general, and the virtue tradition in particular has consistently held that although we can speak about care (usually called "sentiment") as something different from justice, we cannot speak about virtuous or morally right action unless we are speaking about action which is *both* motivated by care and concern, and which is just. Aristotle (third century *B.C.*) and Cicero (second century *B.C.*) are but two of the better known ancient male philosophers whose writings neither excluded nor diminished the importance of care in moral action. Hume, and indeed the entire "virtue" tradition in moral philosophy have stressed the importance of developing sentiments of care and concern for others. Within that tradition, there have been those who, like Hume, emphasized that sentiment plus reason, and not reason alone, was essential for principled action.

Although fourth century *B.C.* Greek women philosophers wrote within a society with distinct gender roles, their writings suggest that they supported a gender undifferentiated moral theory. A superficial reading of these writings by women who were contemporaries of Plato, appears at first to support some aspects of Carol Gilligan's (1982) thesis that when making moral choices, women tend to appeal to "an ethic of care" while men tend to appeal to "an ethic of justice." When we examine the works in context as well as in greater detail, we see that an argument can be sustained that ancient women philosophers viewed both "caring" and "justice" as essential elements of morally right action. In the sections below, I shall show how when read as examples of "social morality" these writings suggest that ancient women philosophers supported a gender difference view and when read as examples of "theoretical morality" (moral philosophy) the works of ancient women philosophers support a gender undifferentiated view of morality.

Social Morality and a Gender Difference View

Surviving correspondence and fragments of larger works by Phintys of Sparta and Perictione I (Waithe 1987b) present the view that women can best fulfill their social roles by preserving harmonious relationships within families, and by raising children to be virtuous. Consider the comments of Phintys of Sparta from Fragment II of *On the Moderation of Women*:

The noblest honor and the chief glory of a married woman is to bring witness of her virtue with respect to her husband through her own children if, haply, they should bear the stamp of likeness to the father who sired them. This sums up the subject of moderation with respect to marriage (Phintys of Sparta, in Waithe 1987, p. 30).

The idea that the virtue of a woman is to care for her husband at the expense of caring for herself, and even at the expense of her own well-being is graphically described by Perictione I:

A woman must bear everything on the part of her husband, even if he should be unfortunate, or fail on account of ignorance or illness or drink, or cohabit with other women. For this error is forgiven in the case of men; for women, never. Rather, retribution is imposed. She must keep the law and not be envious (Perictione I, in Waithe 1987, p. 34).

It is interesting to look at the text of Perictione I *On the Harmony of Women* (Waithe 1987a, pp. 32–34). She addresses what Gilligan would identify as selfishness and shows that what is good is caring for others, and then recommends acceptance of the illogic of the inequality between a woman and her husband. A later philosopher, Theano II, writing to Euboule, urges her friend not to spoil her children: "Hardships, my dear, serve as a hardening-up process for children, a process by which virtue is perfected" (Waithe 1987a, p. 43). This suggests a level of development in which the interdependence of mother and child is acknowledged, and in which spoiling is understood to hurt the child while exploiting the parent's weakness in giving in to the child's demands. (See Meyers and Kittay 1987, pp. 7–8, for a similar description of Gilligan's account of development.)

These writings and other writings by women philosophers of the same period are explicitly about the morality of caring: caring for spouses, babies, servants, slaves, and oneself. These excerpts from the texts describe a social morality in which women's job is to care for others. However, there is a clear distinction between social morality (the norms of society) and theoretical morality (moral philosophy). On the level of social custom, these philosophers acknowledged that the social structure in which they found themselves was one in which "women's work" facilitated "men's work."

In that society, "women's work" of caring for and nurturing the development of persons who would be capable of acting justly was a necessary condition which enabled "men's work": administering the wheels of social justice in the marketplace and in politics. However, other aspects of works from this group give us a glimpse of ancient women philosophers' views about moral theory. I want to suggest that, on a theoretical level, these ancient women philosophers saw no difference between care and justice.

Moral Theory and a Gender Undifferentiated View

When these same works by women philosophers are examined as examples of applied moral theory, a gender undifferentiated position emerges. These ancient women philosophers placed caring in the context of justice. Since the state is composed of households, justice and harmony in the state would be affected by how well women fulfilled their social responsibility to raise just, harmonious children. A surviving fragment from Aesara of Lucania's *Book on Human Nature* provides the key to understanding the philosophic perspective of these writings. Aesara's fragment begins: "Human nature seems to me to provide a standard of law and justice both for the home and for the city" (Aesara of Lucania in Waithe 1987 p. 20). Although Aesara's fragment does not address the question of gender differences in moral decision-making directly, it does clearly indicate that she, and perhaps other women philosophers of that period, held that both the ethic of care (a moral principle acted upon within the home, by women) and the ethic of justice (a moral principle acted upon outside the home, in the public arena of market and court, by men) derived from a theory of human nature. If I am correct in my reading of Aesara's fragment, and if I am correct in thinking that she presents a theoretical perspective shared by other Greek women philosophers of her period, then the writings of those women should be consistent with the view that moral principles are not gender-bound. On this view, an ethic of care is not grounded in "woman's nature," nor is an ethic of justice grounded in "man's nature." Rather, care and justice are equally grounded in "human nature," and it is merely a matter of social convention that women perform care-giving roles and men perform justice-giving roles. These social differences are not natural differences which, like child-bearing roles, are a consequence of biological distinctions between women and men.

Indeed, when we look at the writings by the women philosophers of this period, we see an ethic of care presented as a way of treating others fairly, a way of fulfilling duties voluntarily contracted through marriage, and, as a way of modelling morally virtuous behavior. The letter of Theano II to Kallisto claims that unless a woman is just and harmonious, the household in which she lives cannot be a just and harmonious one (Waithe 1987a, p. 43). Caring is presented as the context in which true justice (as distinct from mere procedural justice) can be rendered. The works of these ancient women suggest to me that they held a particular view of the connection between theoretical morality and social morality. That view appears to be as follows: On the theoretical level, 'care' and 'justice' are mutually dependent moral constructs. Both constructs derive from an ungendered view of *human* moral nature, rather than from separate concepts of *male* and *female* morality. Action is not considered to be moral unless it is both caring and just. There is no evidence that Greek women philosophers considered women to be less capable than men of achieving the moral norm. However, it is generally agreed among historians of that period that most male philosophers held the view that women's souls were not equally capable of virtue.

EVOLUTION OF A SECOND GENDER UNDIFFERENTIATED VIEW

The evolution of a second gender undifferentiated view, the view that both men and women are capable of morality, took many centuries. This evolution consisted of reactions to a complex Christian theological view about salvation. The Christian view was that men, not women, were made "in God's image and likeness," and therefore, only men could be saved. One aspect of being made in God's image and likeness was having the capacity for reason. The church considered that moral behavior which could lead to salvation required the ability to reason, and women were not capable of reason. In the eyes of the church, morality was gendered. The social marginalization of women as caregivers and their exclusion from the arena of social justice (church, market, and state) was validated by Christian moral philosophy. Caring as a moral construct was relegated to a moral emotion, an affective capacity; whereas, justice as a moral construct was elevated to a deliberate moral action, an intellectual capacity to reason about social interactions. In this section, I will (1) describe the general growth and development of aspects of Christian moral philosophy which are relevant to the care/justice issue, and then (2) describe how a second gender undifferentiated view evolved among women philosophers who reacted to Christianity's denial of women's capacity for morality. However, it is important to bear in mind that what I describe as "Christian moral philosophy" gradually became much more than just another moral theory: it came to characterize the values, beliefs, religions, and governments of Western civilization. Women's rejection of certain aspects of "Christian moral philosophy" constituted a rejection of aspects of Western civilization itself.

Christian Moral Philosophy and Care/Justice

During the two to eight centuries which passed from the time Aesara, Perictione I, Theano II, and Perictione II lived, through the development of the early Christian church[3] social roles of women as well as philosophical theories about "women's nature" increasingly marginalized women. The distinctions between social morality and theoretical morality which, I have argued, were understood by earlier women philosophers, appear to have become blurred toward the end of the ancient era. In the early Judeo-Christian era, Christian philosophy portrayed women in moral extremes. During the first five centuries after Christ, views about women's capacity for morality were characterized by the apposition of the two major female personas of the Judeo-Christian tradition, Eve and Mary. Eve was depicted as exploiting Adam's susceptibility to "weakness of the flesh," causing him to allow emotion to override his reason, and to defy the religious authority of a male God. Eve represented all women and was held responsible for the "fall" of man(kind) from the grace of God. (See Ginzburg, 1946, for a fuller account.) Because of Eve, all humans were born in "original sin" which blotted their souls and prevented their salvation. Not only were women dangerous from the point of view of men's salvation, but it was reasonable to question whether women themselves could be saved. Women were depicted as amoral temptresses who seduced rational men to disobey God's law and thereby risk eternal damnation. The message was that, particularly in circumstances of moral decision making, women were dangerous.

However, there was also Mary, the second important female persona. Mary represented the ideal of female virtue (obedience and chastity), and was critical in the salvation of humanity (Theodotus of Ancyra, in Garland 1961). Mary was more than a persona. She was an historical person. It soon became theologically untenable to deny women's capacity for salvation when Christ's own mother was depicted as a virgin who was assumed bodily into heaven. Moreover, it became unthinkable that she who had obediently declared herself to be "the handmaid of the Lord"; she who had chastely given birth[4] to Christ, could have been born in "original sin." With the doctrine of the Immaculate Conception, characterizations of the obedient, submissive,[5] chaste Mary became apposed to those of the disobedient, seductive Eve.

Were women moral, (and Mary the archetype of all women) or were women incapable of morality (and Eve the archetype of all women)? A related question sometimes raised during this period was whether women were capable of meeting a necessary condition for moral action; were women, like lower animals, merely sentient, affective creatures, or did they,

like men, have "rational souls"? The discussion about moral differences
between men and women turned into discussions of whether women had rational souls and were made in the image and likeness of God. This was a
subject of debate, and early Christian philosophers were not in agreement
about the answer. A minority which included Makrina of Neocaesaria (circa
A.D. 300) (Waithe 1987a, pp. 139–168), Clemens of Alexandria, Basil the
Great, and other early Church Fathers, held that women *were* made in
God's image and therefore had rational souls which were capable of the
kind of moral virtue that is important for salvation.

To the extent that justice was perceived to be a "rational" response (and
therefore male and moral), while caring was perceived to be an "affective"
response (and therefore female and nonmoral), the question whether
women had rational souls can be seen as an early version of the care/jus-
tice issue. It should also be remembered that while this debate was taking
place in the early centuries after Christ, the rise of the "Holy Roman Empire" was underway, complete with the repression of "pagan" (i.e.,
Greek) philosophy, and the suppression of scholarly discussion of works
by ancient philosophers. This meant a suppression not only of works of
moral philosophy which fit more squarely in the "justice" tradition (e.g.,
Plato's *Republic*), but those which also fit the "virtue" tradition (e.g.,
Aristotle's *Nicomachean Ethics* VII). During this period many of the
works of ancient philosophers (including perhaps those of the ancient
women philosophers) were deliberately destroyed or removed to far-flung
parts of the Roman Empire, or to distant Arabic centers of learning. Not
only were the distinctions between social and philosophical morality blurred during this time, but access to a philosophic tradition that was relevant
to the discussion of gender differences in moral judgment was largely
denied. The view that women were not capable of rationality, and
therefore, not capable of moral action became firmly rooted in Western
civilization.

However, if women's own writings did not expressly argue for their intellectual (and therefore moral) equality with men, the mere fact that
pagan women philosophers such as Julia Domna and Hypatia of Alexandria had demonstrated their abilities as philosophers provided *argumentum
ad demonstratum*. The perception of Christian women philosophers
became that they had rational souls, and not only rational souls but souls
made in the image and likeness of God. Pagan as well as Christian women
philosophers of this late ancient period believed that they could do more
than exemplify the affective virtues of caring, concern, piety, and obedience. They could exemplify the intellectual virtues of insight,
understanding, analysis, and philosophical argumentation. Women whose
achievements stood in marked contrast to Christian doctrine were considered "masculine" or simply, "exceptions to the rule." It was from the

ranks of those exceptional women that the second version of the gender undifferentiated view would later evolve.

Women Philosophers and a Second Gender Undifferentiated View

In the early middle ages, young girls who were doweried to monasteries
and convents for a life of religious service increasingly had opportunities to
learn Latin. With literacy came opportunities to illuminate and hand copy
the writings of the early Church Fathers. One such woman was Hildegard of
Bingen (1098-1179) (Gossman, in press). Hildegard challenged official
church doctrine on the nature of women's souls, and developed a concept of
women's moral equality with men. Hildegard's moral anthropology considers the woman to be a human being who may be different from man in
temperament, but who is no different in wisdom, moral worth, or moral
capacity.

The medieval philosopher Heloise (1101-1164) (Gilson 1951) was widely
known as an exponent of Cicero's philosophy of love. She argued forcefully
against marriage to Abelard on the grounds that the social constraints of
marriage would kill their highly intellectualized, sensual relationship
(Hamilton, 1966). Love for Abelard convinced her that marriage to him
would be morally wrong: as a married cleric, his authority as a philoso-
pher/theologian would diminish. "Of a certainty we shall both be
destroyed; and our sorrow match in its intensity the love that has been
ours" (Hamilton 1966, p. 42). After the birth of their illegitimate child, and
against her better judgment, she acquiesced to the marriage. Her uncle,
Fulbert, retaliated by having Abelard castrated. In her view, Heloise married in obedience to and out of love for Abelard and was therefore material-
ly but not morally responsible for Fulbert's injustice toward Abelard. Her
action was morally right, she argued, because it was a product of caring:
"In a wicked deed, rectitude of action depends not on the effect of the thing
but on the affections of the agent, not on what is done but with what
dispositions it is done" (Heloisa [1884-1890], in Migne 184).

The renaissance of the early fourteenth century revived an interest in the
rediscovered texts of ancient Greek philosophers. Christine de Pisan
(1365-1431), who was educated at the court of Charles V, was among those
women who gained access to ancient philosophy. Pisan offered arguments
against the inferiority and subordination of women based on her own view
of social justice. Her *Cité des Dames* (Pisan 1982) constructs a walled city
for the protection of women from physical as well as moral harm. In her
city, it is the female "rational" or "moral" virtues, Ladies Reason, Justice,
and Duty, rather than the nurturant virtues, which guide women. Through
the voice of these rational virtues, Pisan argued that the oppression of

women was contrary to the goal of improving society itself. Interestingly, Pisan said that women whose activities are limited by specific social roles should work hard to avoid the kinds of activities that dull their intellect and sap their strength to the detriment of the common social good.

In the early part of the modern period, the civil state replaced the church as the primary source of political authority. State persecution of religious minorities resulted in massive emigrations to the New World and rapid global colonization by European powers. Even as European nations reduced colonized populations to slavery or indenture, commerce with non-white races created new sensitivities in many Europeans to the moral equality of all races and of both genders. Conventional social morality of the early modern period characterized women as caregivers who were capable only of affective, emotional response, and characterized men as administrators of justice who were capable of highly intellectual, reasoned decisions. The question whether women were made in God's image and likeness and were capable of salvation had long faded. However, the care/justice issue continued to be expressed as the same debate over women's capacity for reason which had characterized the early church. Conventional social morality continued to permit unequal social treatment of women, and justified female social inequality by appeals to claims that women were physically and intellectually inferior to males. Although Aesara of Lucania (Waithe 1987b) had long ago observed that "human nature" provided the standard for judging the morality of actions, some philosophers of the enlightenment period were now also beginning to address theories of human moral equality. They inquired whether all *humans* were created morally equal, and whether human nature indeed provided a standard for judging the morality of individual actions as well as the morality of social policy.

It is within this context that women philosophers became advocates for equal social treatment for women. Some, like the Spanish philosopher Oliva Sabuco de Nantes Barerra turned to a more inclusive focus on the concept of *human* nature (Sabuco de Nantes, 1888). In 1585 she described her view of human nature as incomplete without both the capacity for emotional attachment and the capacity for reasoned justice. Other women philosophers argued in support of equal social rights for women by arguing that there was no natural intellectual inequality between men and women; we are all humans. For example, the French philosopher Marie le Jars de Gournay (1565–1645) (Zedler, in press) disputed the received doctrine of the natural inferiority of women to men. Rather than portray women as inferior in their capacity for morality, Gournay's *Egalité des hommes et des femmes* (1622) argued for their equality. In her view, gender was not part of the essence of human nature. Gender differentiation was necessary only for reproduction; men and women are intellectual and moral equals. In *Grièf des dames* (1626) she argued for social equality of the sexes.

The seventeenth-century Dutch philosopher Anna Maria van Schurmann (1607–1678) wrote *The learned maid, or whether a maid may be a schollar?* (1659). The argument of her book was in the form of a classical logic proof with premises leading to the conclusion that women are rational and are fully capable of being philosophers. The Mexican philosopher Sor Juana In` es de la Cruz (1648–1695) (Morkovsky, in press) held views on personal liberation and the education of women which suggest that she also did not consider care and justice to be separable criteria of ethical action. Although her writing was primarily in the area of epistemology, Damaris Masham (1659–1708) (Frankel, in press) objected not only to the denial of educational opportunities to most women, but to the double standard of morality imposed on women, particularly regarding chastity.

With the publication in 1790 of *A Vindication of the Rights of Man* and in 1792 of *A Vindication of the Rights of Woman* (which was a response to Thomas Paine's *Rights of Man*) Mary Wollstonecraft's (Lindemann, in press) claim that women were the moral and intellectual equals of men led to widespread political debate. Wollstonecraft not only argued for women's moral equality, but insisted that the failure of men and of the society controlled by men to acknowledge women's equality was itself an injustice. In a very forceful way, the circularity of the prevailing views on women's morality was used by Wollstonecraft to argue that men, who claimed to have a monopoly on reason and, therefore, on the capacity to administer justice, acted unjustly in exercising that monopoly.

Like many of her contemporaries,[6] nineteenth-century feminist philosopher Harriet Taylor Mill (Waithe, in press b) considered the gender difference issue insulting. Instead, she argued for women's equal rights. In an essay on sex equality (Taylor 1970) she argued that women were intellectually capable and morally competent for employment in any profession. Frenchwoman Clarisse Coignet (b. 1823) (Allen, in press) also argued for women's moral equality. A Kantian philosopher, she argued that women ought to be considered sovereign ends in themselves. Viewing both genders as having equal capacities for justice and caring need not destroy the family, she said; rather, such a perspective could form the cornerstone of the family unit.

The arguments of philosophers like Mary Wollstonecraft, Harriet Taylor Mill, and Clarisse Coignet represent somewhat of a departure from the long tradition which had supported social inequalities between men and women. These philosophers simply denied that there were relevant differences between men's and women's abilities to reason. This denial was made without challenging the traditional justice framework which associated justice with the capacity for reason. In their view, intellectual equality implied that both men and women were capable of justice. And if both were capable of justice, men would lack any justification for denying equal social rights to women. But it is Clemence Royer (1830–1892) (Waithe, in press b) who might be considered a modern proponent of the ancient view that care and justice are mutually dependent theoretical moral constructs. Royer (1881) argued that societies which seek to become truly just must support the growth of those social institutions which foster the development of humanistic concern. While her contemporaries argued that men and women do not differ in their capacity for rationality, Royer claimed that social morality must be based on a moral theory which holds that care and justice are mutually dependent theoretical constructs.

THE THIRD VERSION: NATURAL DIFFERENCES ARE NOT MORALLY SIGNIFICANT

Not all women philosophers of the modern period followed in the tradition of the medieval and modern women philosophers who held that women's capacity for reason was equal to that of men. Indeed, philosophers Bathsua Pell Makin, Margaret Cavendish, and Antoinette Brown Blackwell held that there *were* differences between men and women regarding both the capacity for reason and the capacity for care. However, each argued that the differences were not morally significant and could not justify differential treatment of women. In their views, women and men may have different capacities for reason, and different dispositions to care and to nurture, but that did not justify a more restrictive range of rights for women than for men.

Englishwoman Bathsua Pell Makin (b. 1612), (Waithe, in press b) was one of the earliest proponents of this position. In her *Essay to Revive the Ancient Education of Gentlewomen* (Makin 1980), Makin argued that women who had been viewed as prodigious intellects were models to which many women could aspire. To garner government support for a women's college, she argued that the education of women would even contribute to their abilities to fulfill their socially ordained roles as caregivers. At the same time, she argued forcefully for women's economic rights to control of their own finances. English philosopher Margaret Cavendish (1617/23–1673) (Schiebinger, in press) called for what she considered to be the masculization of women. Women, she argued, should have much more than physical and intellectual prowess. In her view, women could be the moral superiors of men if they cultivated reason without sacrificing the "feminine" virtues of temperance, humility, patience, chastity, piety, and modesty. The American philosopher/theologian, Antoinette Brown Blackwell (1825–1921) (Murphy, in press) also held the view that women's morality was different from men's and was to be valued because of that difference, that is, women brought compassion to justice, and caring to rights.

Blackwell argued that women were every bit as inductive as men were deductive, but that both forms of reasoning were of equal importance. In her view, men and women were equally capable of care and love, although women excelled in nurturance of others.

CONCLUSIONS

The historical discussion of whether there are differences between care and justice, whether there are gender differences in the capacity for moral judgment, and whether there are different predispositions toward caring or toward justice, began more than 2,000 years ago. Indeed, three versions of a gender undifferentiated view have occupied the writings of women philosophers during that period. One version was that care and justice were mutually dependent theoretical constructs. A second version was that women were capable of morality. This version of the gender undifferentiated view first asserted that women had souls, and later, that women had rational souls. A third version of the gender undifferentiated view emerged more recently. According to this version, there were *morally insignificant* gender differences in natural capacity for, or natural disposition toward care or justice. Women philosophers who expressly argued for this view included forceful advocates of women's equal rights. In their view women ought not have fewer rights under the law merely because they are more caring than men, or tend to prefer inductive reasoning to deductive reasoning.

In this century, Carol Gilligan (1982; 1987), Nell Noddings (1984; this volume), Jane Roland Martin (1985; this volume), and Sara Ruddick (1984) have been among the most vocal critics of the "justice orientation" of Kohlberg's moral psychology, which has its primary origins in moral philosophy of the last three centuries. Now, contemporary theorists have an opportunity to continue the historical debate by reconsidering not only the views of Hume and other male proponents of the virtue tradition, but also the views of earlier women philosophers. How can we best move the gender differences debate forward? We can begin by reassessing the contributions of past women philosophers to that debate. We can examine whether moral action requires that one care about relationships among individuals. We can investigate whether action that does not require the actor to reason well about preserving caring relationships ought to be called moral action. We can inquire whether morality requires that one be committed to acting justly toward those for whom one cannot care, and toward those with whom caring relationships have not yet developed. Lastly, we can seek to determine whether the virtue and justice traditions within moral philosophy can be synthesized within a gender undifferentiated philosophy of human morality.

NOTES

1. According to Plato, *Timeaus* 42c., the soul of an unvirtuous man is reincarnated as a woman or as an animal.

2. Some may consider Nietzsche and Kant to be exceptions to this view. I am not prepared to address that argument here.

3. Although most of the evidence indicates that these philosophers were contemporaries of Plato (428–337 *B.C.*) or of Aristotle (384–322 *B.C.*), some evidence suggests that they may have lived as late as *circa* 100 *B.C.*

4. According to Wolfskeel (1987), Mary's virginity was first declared in the Council of Ephesus, in *A.D.* 431.

5. Wolfskeel (1987) indicates that the natural submissiveness of all women was upheld by the Synod of Gangra, fourth century.

6. For example, Harriet Martineau and Eliza Flower.

REFERENCES

Aesara of Lucania. (1987). Book on human nature. Translated by V. L. Harper. *In A history of women philosophers*, Vol. 1, ed. M. E. Waithe. Dordrecht: Martinus Nijhoff Publishers.

Allen, J. (In press). Clarisse Coignet. In *A history of women philosophers*, Vol. 3, ed. M. E. Waithe. Dordrecht: Martinus Nijhoff Publishers.

Aristotle. *Ethica Nicomachea*.

Baier, A. C. (1987). Hume, The women's moral theorist? In *Women and moral theory*, ed. E. F. Kittay and D. T. Meyers. Totowa, NJ: Rowman & Littlefield.

Frankel, L. (In press). Damaris Cudworth Masham. In *A history of women philosophers*, Vol. 3, ed. M. E. Waithe. Dordrecht: Martinus Nijhoff Publishers.

Gilligan, C. (1982). *In a different voice: Psychological theory and women's development*. Cambridge, MA: Harvard University Press.

———. (1987). Moral orientation and moral development. In *Women and Moral Theory*, ed. E. F. Kittay and D. T. Meyers. Totowa, NJ: Rowman & Littlefield.

Gilson, E. (1951). *Héloise and Abélard*. L. K. Shook authorized translation of *Héloise et Abélard*. Chicago: Henry Regnery Co.

Ginzburg, L. (1946). *The legends of the Jews*. Philadelphia: The Jewish Publication Society of America.

Gossman, E. (In press). Hildegard of Bingen. In *A history of women philosophers,* Vol. 2, ed. M. E. Waithe. Dordrecht: Martinus Nijhoff Publishers.

Hamilton, E. (1966). *Heloise*. London: Hodder and Stoughton.

Heloisa. (1844–1890). *Heloissae Epistolae*, 184. In *Tatrologiae cursus colcumpletus*, series graeca, series latina, ed. Migne. Paris: Garnieri Fratres.

Lindemann, K. (In press). Mary Wollstonecraft. In *A history of women philosophers*, Vol. 3, ed. M. E. Waithe. Dordrecht: Martinus Nijhoff Publishers.

Makin, B. (1980). *Essay to revive the ancient education of gentlewomen*. Reprint by the Augustan Reprint Society, Publication Number 202. LA: University of California Williams Andrew Clark Library.

Martin, J. (1985) *Reclaiming a conversation*. New Haven, CT: Yale University Press.

Meyers, D. T., and Kittay, E., eds. (1987). Introduction. In *Women and moral theory*. Totowa NJ: Rowman & Littlefield.

Morkovsky, M. C. (in press). Sor Juana Inèz de la Cruz. In *A history of women philosophers*, Vol. 2, ed. M. E. Waithe. Dordrecht: Martinus Nijhoff Publishers.

Murphy, J. S. (In press). Antoinette Brown Blackwell. In *A history of women philosophers*, Vol. 3, ed. M. E. Waithe. Dordrecht: Martinus Nijhoff Publishers.

Noddings, N. (1984). *Caring: A feminine approach to ethics and moral education*. Berkeley, CA: University of California Press.

Perictione I. On the harmony of women. Translated by V. L. Harper. In *A history of women philosophers*. Vol. 1, ed. M. E. Waithe. Dordrecht: Martinus Nijhoff Publishers.

Phintys of Sparta. (1987). On the moderation of women. Translated by V. L. Harper. In *A history of women philosophers*. Vol. 1, ed. M. E. Waithe. Dordrecht: Martinus Nijhoff Publishers.

de Pisan, C. (1982). *The book of the city of ladies*. Translated by E. J. Richards. New York: Persea.

Plato. *Timeaus*. 42c.

Royer, C. (1881). *Le bien et la loi morale; éthique et téléologie*. Paris: Guillaumin et Cie.

Ruddick, S. (1984). Maternal thinking. In *Mothering*, ed. J. Treblicot. Totowa, NJ: Rowman and Allenheld.

Sabuco de Nantes, O. (1888). Nueva filosofía de la naturaleza del hombre. In *Sabuco de Nantes Obras*, ed. O. Cuartero. Madrid: Ricardo Fé.

Schiebinger, L. (In press). Margaret Cavendish. In *A history of women philosophers*, Vol. 3, ed. M. E. Waithe. Dordrecht: Martinus Nijhoff Publishing.

van Schurmann, A. M. (1659). *The learned maid, or whether a maid may be a scholler?* London: Redmayne.

Taylor, H. (1970). Untitled essay. In *Essays on sex equality: John Stuart Mill and Harriet Taylor Mill*, ed. A. Rossi. Chicago & London: University of Chicago Press.

Theodotus of Ancyra. (1961). Homilia on the state of the Mother of God. In *Acta Concilia Ephesus*, Tome IX, ed. Garland. Paris: Garland.

Waithe, M. E., ed. (1987a). *A history of women philosophers*, Vol. 1. Dordrecht: Martinus Nijhoff Publishers.

Waithe, M. E. (1987b). Late Pythagoreans: Aesara of Lucania, Phintys of Sparta and Perictione I. In *A history of women philosophers*, Vol. 1, ed. M. E. Waithe. Dordrecht: Martinus Nijhoff Publishers.

Waithe, M. E., ed. (In press a). *A history of women philosophers,* Vol. 2. Dordrecht: Martinus Nijhoff Publishers.

———. (In press b). *A history of women philosophers*, Vol. 3. Dordrecht: Martinus Nijhoff Publishers.

Wolfskeel, C. W. (1987). Makrina. In *A history of women philosophers*, Vol. 1, ed. M. E. Waithe. Dordrecht: Martinus Nijhoff Publishers.
Zedler, B. (In press). Marie le Jars de Gournay. In *A history of women philosophers,* Vol. 2, ed. M. E. Waithe. Dordrecht: Martinus Nijhoff Publishers.

2

The Liberation of Caring:
A Different Voice for Gilligan's
"Different Voice"

Bill Puka

A compelling vision of "caring" and its role in women's development has evolved in psychology and gender studies (e.g., Miller 1976; Chodorow 1978; Gilligan 1982; Noddings 1984). Gilligan's "different voice" conception of "care" as an ethical orientation and its contrast to the patriarchal preference for individual rights and justice has had a powerful impact on many fields, including philosophy, and has garnered an enthusiastic international following.

Many of Gilligan's supporters, however, are careful to note the formative nature of her account and its potential dangers. As some put it, Gilligan has helped show that there is some gender difference here, centered around the relational and nuturant orientations of women. Now we must clarify what it is. (Gilligan sometimes qualifies her own views similarly; see Gilligan [1982] pp. 3, 126). Feminist analysis warns that attempting to distinguish woman's caretaking strengths from her socialized, servile weaknesses flirts with sexism itself. It runs the risk of transforming victimization into virtue by merely saying it is so, of legitimizing subjugation to gender in a misguided attempt at self-affirmation. This seems a typical pitfall for oppressed groups, especially in "personal consciousness-raising" approaches to liberation.

In this chapter, I will pose a different voice for Gilligan's "different voice," an alternative hypothesis of what the caring difference might be. On this hypothesis care is not primarily a general course of moral development, but a set of coping strategies for dealing with sexist oppression in particular. In the spirit of care, this hypothesis is designed to "satisfy everyone," including proponents and critics on each side. Foremost, it seeks to preserve care's strengths and the strengths of women's development. Yet in doing so, it pares back some of care's presumed critical relevance to "justice theories" of development, making room for their virtues while deflecting much unnecessary controversy, detrimental to care.[1] The alternative hypothesis also seeks to affirm feminist worries regarding care without threatening Gilligan's main insights or care's research potential.

THE TWO ALTERNATIVES

The First Alternative: Care as Moral Development: Gilligan's Voice

Gilligan (1982) portrays care as both a general orientation toward moral problems (interpersonal problems) and a track of moral development. As an orientation or focus, care expresses an empathetic sense of connectedness to others, of being in-relation with them, actually or potentially. As a track of development, care evolves from an egocentric form of self-care, through a more conventional sort of do-gooder care. It moves on, finally, to a self-chosen, self-reflective, and self-affirming form of mature caring (Gilligan 1982, chaps. 3, 4).

At level 1 of this development, care is self-concerned and self-protective out of a sense of vulnerability. The caring individual seeks above all to avoid hurt and insure psychological survival. With increasing self-confidence and a sense of competence to relate effectively, she sees this protective orientation as selfish and irresponsible. Care then evolves into a more conventional form of caring for others that is socially effective in its adherence to accepted norms. At this second level, the caring person seeks the support and approval of others by living up to their expectations and serving their needs altruistically. On the one hand, this leads to psychological denial and the rationalization of care's slavishness, according to Gilligan. On the other, it breeds a conflicting sense of being put upon and of allowing it to happen, of using the guise of altruism and martyrdom to mask indirect self-interest. With the confidence to face this conflict, and oneself, however, the caring individual moves to level 3. Here she recognizes that self-concern is self-responsible , that an adult must balance care for others with care for self as the contexts of her various relationship require.

At both transition points in the sequence, crises of vulnerability can lead to nihilism and despair, confusion and retreat from care, rather than development. That is, women progress and regress in care, rather than following an invariant, progressive sequence.

Care is defined by theme rather than gender, according to Gilligan (1982, p. 2; 1986). Yet care also is the dominant, spontaneous expression of a "relational social perspective." Since a relational perspective arises spontaneously from the formation of female gender identity and role, care will be the female ethic of choice. (Males characteristically evolve a "separational" or individualistic social perspective, by contrast, and prefer a rights and justice ethic.) In addition, since the most prominent theories of moral development favor the theme of justice, since they "listen to male voices" primarily, these theories tend to discriminate against female development. They underrepresent, distort, and undervalue its "different voice" of caring (Gilligan 1982, chaps. 3, 4). (All references will be from Gilligan's (1982) book unless otherwise indicated.)

The Second Alternative: Care as Subjugation and Liberation

The alternative "care as liberation" hypothesis portrays care primarily as a sexist service orientation, prominent in the patriarchal socialization, social conventions, and roles of many cultures. This care theme is seen best at Gilligan's level 2 which is dominated by "stereotypical feminine virtues" such as "gentleness and tact," and an overriding desire "not to hurt" or disappoint anyone, as Gilligan puts it (pp. 76, 65). Here women "seek survival by trying to satisfy male expectations and find male approval in hopes of male support" (pp. 66-67, 72, 78).

On the liberation hypothesis, the focus of such a care theme can be adjusted by adult women to handle crises of hurt, domination, and rejection usually brought on by males in women's daily lives and relationships as clearly reflected in Gilligan's key studies (pp. 2, 3). Such crises engender various responses, each of which has pros and cons. Care "development" or care *levels* then, actually represent circumscribed coping strategies, of special use to women for facing crises of sexism. While these strategies may be ordered by coping effectiveness, they do not evolve from each other developmentally for the most part. They do not represent general systems of moral competence of the sort that cognitive stages do in classic theories of moral development.

Let us reconsider Gilligan's three levels of care through the lens of this alternative hypothesis. Care at level 1 now becomes primarily a coping strategy for facing hurtful rejection and domination, not for orienting to moral issues generally. It copes with its context, sensibly, by "seeking survival" through self-protection (pp. 75-76, 110-111). Yet the ineffectiveness of this strategy, its "sense of isolation, aloneness, powerlessness," as Gilligan puts it, can often lead to resuming the conventional, slavish approach of level 2 care. In Gilligan's research, such coping requires psychological denial and rationalization when used as a strategy adopted by adult women (pp. 80-85). Level 2's slavishness is especially difficult to live with if one has reflected at all on one's role and treatment in sexist relationships as

Gilligan's respondents have. We would not expect this reflective conflict to arise in the well-socialized girl.

To deal with these inner conflicts of level 2 coping, while facing additional domination and rejection by men, various strategies recommend themselves. Level 3, where the balance between care for others and care for self is struck, is not the obvious alternative. One might revert to level 1, self-protectiveness again. Gilligan describes an assertive model of this strategy which involves "deliberate isolation." Here one sees oneself as "a loner" who is self-sufficient and unfettered to a degree (pp. 75, 89). This form of self-protection would be especially effective in dealing with "level 2" aversion to slavish care and internal level 1 problems of powerlessness and isolation. Yet in addressing these problems in this way, one identifies with one's victimization retreat from care, mistaking it as one's self-affirming strength.

A like strategy of "care" would involve what Gilligan terms "moral nihilism" (pp. 123-126). In its less despairing form, it is a more affirmative approach to self-interest than self-protection is—if nothing is really right or wrong, then "why care? why not be selfish?"

Of course, one may not have the self-confidence for such self-affirmation, not the luck of finding those modes of self-affirmation that "work for you." In this context, one may fall into moral confusion and hopelessness. Gilligan describes this "development" as well—"I'm still in love with him, no matter what he has done, and that really confuses me . . . I can't get him out of my mind" (p. 124). Such regression in caring can also result from the servile strategy of trying level 2 "service orientation" over and over again, despite its failure. Gilligan terms these sorts of phenomena "cycles of repetition" and the "psychology of passivity," though she does not apply these descriptions to level 2.

(When considering the basis of this reinterpretation thus far, three features of Gilligan's account are key. First, care is depicted as progressing and regressing, alternately, not necessarily as evolving in order of levels. Second, Gilligan does not claim, nor offer evidence, that lower levels of care generally occur earlier in development. And finally, Gilligan's studies do not observe any one respondent traversing all three levels of care in order, or otherwise. Therefore, the seemingly undevelopmental disorder or variability of care fits here.)

There are, however, more effective coping strategies that care might try. Through the self-confidence gained by surviving abandonments and hurt, and reflectively learning their lessons, level 3 care may emerge. In this explicit "consciousness-raising" strategy, a woman seeks the "middle path" between self-protection and slavishness. She balances self care with care for others more evenly. Level 3 care is clearly a more subtle and effective path than level 2 coping for confronting the sexist realities a woman faces. It shows significant insight into the validity of benevolent virtues and compassionate responses, along with acknowledgment of their dangers. Here a woman learns where she can exercise her strengths, interests, and commitments within the male power structure and where she would do better to comply with that structure. A delicate contextual balance must be struck to be effective here.

Since this approach carries forward some of the aversive "service orientation" of level 2, its internal effectiveness is enhanced by rationalization, as it was at level 2. Likewise, since the slavishness of this orientation is now more reflectively recognized than at level 2, effective rationalization must take a far more reflective and legitimating form. Thus in this level 3 coping strategy, a woman takes personal responsibility for compliance. She portrays it as adult and self-chosen *in its selectivity*, and even virtuous in this selectivity. Furthermore, she abstracts and generalizes the strategy as a legitimate and even preferred ethic—a carefully balanced, caring-for-others-in-general ethic—from which males could learn much. She distinguishes such a service orientation from slavish level 2 conventionalism by recasting the *limits* of her social and moral power as the very *power* to be limited, to be tentative, contextual, and morally balanced in her exercise of power. Gilligan emphasizes the peculiar virtues of such contextualism and tentativeness in level 3 care (pp. 54-55, 95, 100-102, 165-167).

Partial Developments

As should be apparent, support for this alternative "different voice" will derive from Gilligan's own text. The "care as liberation" hypothesis proposes that Gilligan's observations and *interpretations* of care *may* not best support her overall position that care constitutes moral development. At the least, they lend comparable support to the view that care is primarily a form of coping with sexism. Before we detail this support, a few reflections on the significance of this hypothesis are in order. We will begin with its relation to Gilligan's conception of moral maturity, to possible (sexist) biases in her interpretive theorizing, and to the nondevelopmental strengths of care she uncovers.

While the highest level for care shows a degree of cognitive liberation from sexist oppression, its consciousness-raising may not see through many sexist aspects of its own ethic. In this regard it is morally defective and incomplete rather than mature or adequate. Level 3 care does not accurately identify the causes of its "sense of service" in the sexist nature of social institutions and sexual politics primarily. Rather it "progressively" personalizes and legitimizes responsibility for this orientation as a desirable form of "taking control of one's life" and "taking responsibility for one-self," of learning to feel "adult" and "good about oneself" (e.g., pp. 76-78, 82-85, 91-94).

Unfortunately, Gilligan's descriptions of care maturity at level 3 appear to reflect and legitimate this process. They portray only the effectiveness of care, not the inadequacies of self-alienation involved. These descriptions actually may compound the problem by portraying care's consciousness-raising approach to liberation as a *spontaneous* or *natural* development reflective of female gender. By making this approach dependent on *personal* confidence, psychological *self*-awareness, and on moral *self*-control and *self*-responsibility, Gilligan seemingly weakens the key connection her account draws between relational orientation and female gender identity.

In an account of care's progressive struggle with sexism, level 3 care might be faulted for its lack of political sense or institutional focus out of which a sense of solidarity with other women and a need for cooperative social action might derive. Care's almost total lack of social-institutional focus at level 3 certainly raises questions about its general moral adequacy. The attempt to balance serving others with self care at level 3 does not solve the problem of slavishness. It merely tempers and accommodates to it in a morally questionable way. This accommodation is then intellectualized, especially in Gilligan's descriptions of level 3, by being portrayed as a necessary complement to "male-oriented" justice (p. 100). (Marx described a similar tendency of crude communism to *universalize* private [alienated] property, including women as male property, in a misguided hope of moralizing it.) By contrast, a truly liberated ethic for women (and other oppressed groups) might speak in a truly new voice, expressing themes of unfolding, liberated experience. In so doing it might not promote either responses or demands for individual rights in themselves or in combination. (This perspective on care addresses feminist concerns and those of critical theorists. Obviously it is framed primarily from the perspective of socialist feminism though it hopes to accommodate radical and liberal feminists perspectives as well in the particular context it addresses.)

At the same time, there can be no doubt that it is psychologically and morally better for women to cope with oppression in these caring ways than not at all. To be able to handle a circumscribed range of moral problems through a particular set or orientational strategies surely shows moral skill. Coming to certain valid moral beliefs and insights, working out one's caring stance on key interpersonal situations clearly, represents a moral advance in some cognitive-psychological domain. And of course, it is morally better that people see through oppression part way than not at all. This is true even when they deceive themselves when doing so; after all, self-deception is a skill of sorts in certain contexts. When such moral progress is accompanied by increased self-awareness and confidence, by learning to take control of one's life and responsibility for oneself, additional moral progress is likely to result. These are all moral developments in women's conceptual orientations which Gilligan has uncovered perceptively and ordered artfully. Gilligan has detailed women's moral *socialization* well also, it appears.

Still, the evolution from somewhat duped and debilitated in some domain to somewhat disabused and functional in that particular domain differs from steadily progressive development in general competence. In this latter process we primarily move from fairly competent to progressively more so. Circumscribed moral coping skills tailored to gender-specific and oppressive contexts differ from broad systems of cognitive moral competence. Such systems organize and process the fundamentals of social experience for all, at the most basic level, while recognizing that much of our most salient experience is not of this sort.

Theories of human development in moral cognition, such as those of Piaget and Kohlberg, seek to chart the progression of such basic meaning and reasoning systems. As a result, care coping and its struggle for liberation need not be covered by the classic theories of moral development which Gilligan criticizes. Nor do these theories discriminate against care when leaving out such phenomena. Likewise, such theories need not, and should not, cover the so-called "justice focus" that Gilligan associates with male gender preferences, nor should it cover any other "macho" ethic there may be. This is so even when such orientations primarily speak to male experience and reflect patriarchal competences in sexist society.

The theories of Piaget, Kohlberg, and especially Freud should be criticized for *bias*, patriarchal and otherwise. However, where justice bias in basic cognitive *structure* is found, it will not likely *discriminate* against care *orientation*, as Gilligan describes this phenomenon. And when such biases are removed, such caring is not likely to be better represented in these sorts of human developmental theories.

"Slave Morality" and Other Ideologies

To avoid misunderstanding, a few brief reflections on the underlying assumptions of this analysis are needed. The "care as liberation" hypothesis utilizes the speculative conceptual models and political jargon of critical theory for two reasons. First, it seeks to emphasize the uncanny relationship between care maturity, as Gilligan portrays it, and the "slave morality" phenomenon long recognized in this tradition. Second, it seeks to show how Gilligan's own critical approach to exposing patriarchy in classic moral development theory might apply to her own view. It does this, in part, by applying the sort of analysis Gilligan offers of level 2 caring to her level 3 caring.

Gilligan's critique, after all, tries to show how males "rationalize" their gender-identity needs through moral (justice) orientations. They claim such needs as their just due. Patriarchal theories then further "rationalize" this rationalization by abstracting and legitimizing it at its "highest" level as a generally applicable form of moral competence. The "care as liberation" hypothesis builds on Gilligan's own observations of how women rationalize their moral victimization at level 2. It suggests how care theory may further "rationalize" this circumscribed sort of rationalization by abstracting and legitimizing it (at its "highest" level) as a generally applicable form of moral competence. In offering this analysis I do not assume that women or victims of oppression generally suffer more "ideological distortion" *overall* than those who oppress them, far from it. Rather this analysis posits partial distortions of one sort, in relation to one sort of coping, and only to a degree.

The "slave morality" phenomenon, as we know, was identified most vividly in the spread of Christianity among poor and oppressed peoples. As Nietzscheans observed, for example, the Christian message of "love as service" appeals by transforming vices of subservience into virtues of redemption. "Bear your cross, be humble, meek, patient, and long suffering for His sake. Love and give even to those who abuse you, asking nothing for yourself, and all will be given to you." Such a message appeals even more when it prescribes such virtues and distributes such burdens to all, as is especially notable in Christianity. Marx identified this ideological "opiate" in secular ideals as well, including ideals of communism. As noted, he predicted that proletarians, victimized by private property, would misconceive their liberation in the ideology of equal property, equal distribution of wealth. In this way they would at least share their victimization "after the revolution." For Marx, Nietzsche, and others, truly liberating moral revolution (or development) is not found in such selective validation of servitude as one climbs out of it. It does not consist in balancing or equalizing servitude. Rather, moral adequacy is found in a radical transformation of our understanding of human welfare and mutuality. Of course, this transformation need not overturn enduring virtues of the Feminine, noted by radical feminists and Gilligan as well.

It is a defining feature of slave moralities, whether posed by male Brahmin in Hinduism, orthodox Jews in early Christianity, or gentlemanly Aristocrats in Confucianism, that duty, obligation, and response-ability define what is right and good. Assertive claims, rights, or merits are barely visible. Insofar as care accommodates rights (Gilligan 1982, chap. 5) it also construes them as obligations (to self) and *must* accord them secondary, if not tertiary status.

While the "care as liberation" hypothesis is not dependent on such speculative positions, nor the often slanted or overgeneralized observations that accompany them, it benefits from what commonsense plausibility they have.[2] (See Nicholson [1983] for a very interesting analysis in a related tradition.)

It is important to recognize, however, that challenges to the moral and psychological adequacy of care and coping, from a critical theory perspective, are somewhat secondary to the intent of this hypothesis. The "slave morality" analysis applies only to one aspect of the "consciousness-raising" component of level 3 care. The heart of "care as liberation" distinguishes care as socialization and skillful coping from care as general moral development. In this way, as noted, it preserves many of care's psychological strengths while fending off damaging counter-criticisms from classic theories of moral development. There is no dispute, I take it, that Gilligan's contrast between care and justice, female relationality and male individuation, captures gender *socialization* by and large. Nor is there likely to be dispute that effective coping, for either gender, *might* vary these themes in ways that Gilligan's care levels depict. Rather the current Kohlberg-Gilligan dispute, for example, is over whether these themes spontaneously evolve in a way that expresses holistic cognitive systems and their inherent processes of constructional self-transformation. Care need not enter this cognitive-developmental domain, nor theoretical controversy, to make its contribution.

It also is important to recognize that the explicitly feminist analysis of care coping I offered here, while important in its own right, may be one aspect of a broader view concerning "response to authoritarianism." Care levels bear a strong resemblance to patterns of attitudinal assimilation and accomodation commonly observed among poor and oppressed groups, or in oppressive situations. Taking the levels in order, their "oppressive focus" may be rendered in commonsense terms: Level 1—protect yourself against harm from those in power. Ensure your psychological survival in the face of ongoing domination through strategies of self-protection and self-concern. Level 2—To overcome ongoing powerlessness, play the roles those in power set for you. Serve and sacrifice to gain their approval and support, thereby participating in their power and avoiding harm. Be circumspect in pursing your true interests, or even in recognizing them; maintain a sense of fulfillment and self-esteem in expressing the competences of pragmatic services. Level 3—With the partial success of strategy 2, and where otherwise possible, acknowledge your (nonthreatening) true interests. Ferret out spheres of power for pursuing them within gaps of the established power structure. Embrace the competences of those oppressed roles one cannot avoid. Identify with them and use them with one's "true" competences as a source of evolving strength and pride.

Social scientists have observed this sort of pattern in the orientation of inmates in prison camps as associated with a related phenomenon, "identification with the aggressor" (e.g., Bettleheim 1943; A. Freud 1946; Sanford 1955). Kohlberg has observed it in the prison communities he has studied (Kohlberg, Kaufman and Scharf 1975; Jennings and Kohlberg 1983; Jennings , Killkenny, and Kohlberg 1983). There also are anecdotal accounts (novels, films, documentaries) of this pattern in blue-collar orientations toward authoritarian management and in Third World orientations toward the "economic imperialism" of industrialized nations. The pattern of response may not always unfold in order, nor need each strategy be tried by each "inmate". But then, neither does care unfold in order, according to Gilligan. Nor has Gilligan observed all levels of care in the development of any one respondent.

In this context, it is notable that Gilligan portrayed care levels only in the responses of women facing the oppressive machinations of sexist institutions and relationships (pp. 71-72, 107-108). In particular, Gilligan's respondents faced threats of male rejection and abandonment in love relationships due to unexpected pregnancies. They consciously saw their abortion decisions as severe crises for these relationships and themselves.

Again, the "care as liberation" hypothesis is not dependent on the sort of global and anecdotal observations cited above, though it benefits from their strongest and most shared insights. This hypothesis can and will be supported from Gilligan's own account of care and its relation to the field of moral development.

WORKING HYPOTHESIS

Since "care as liberation" is a working hypothesis designed for comparison with Gilligan's "different voice" interpretation of findings, its supporting case must be framed relative to Gilligan's as well. It must "argue" that Gilligan studies (1) socialization, reflective consciousness-raising, and coping more than moral development, (2) gender-based coping more than a care theme of coping which women happen to prefer, and (3) coping with oppression and especially sexism rather than more general coping with moral issues. The fact that this hypothesis derives its case from Gilligan's own text reflects Gilligan's own acknowledgment that care is influenced by socialization and coping with sexism. As noted, however, her account opts for the dominance of moral developmental processes in care's evolution, viewing other factors as secondary. This may be a function of the Kohlbergian framework from which her work stems. The "care as liberation" hypothesis questions this interpretation based on the nature of Gilligan's reported observations and research methods. Thus, while it poses themes for care, it does so in Gilligan's own voice. (It is best thought of as part of an internal debate which Gilligan might have with herself, or which supporters might have among themselves, regarding how to voice the caring they hear.) We begin with points (2) and (3) above.

Women and Sexism

It is easy to misunderstand Gilligan's claim that the "different voice" is characterized by theme, not gender (Gilligan 1986). Care is not a theme that all women must prefer, or that all women have been observed preferring. Neither is it a theme males cannot adopt. However, it is the theme that Gilligan considers characteristic of women, not men. This is so, in the first instance, because Gilligan claims to have found an "empirical association" of this sort. But more important, it is so because Gilligan claims to have identified the apparent cause of this association, the relational orientation built into female gender-identity. Gilligan's research is aimed at uncovering this distinctively gender-based relation. Likewise, her research with colleagues and students is focused on the gender difference issue (Lyons 1983; Langdale 1983; Johnston 1985).

> The different voice I describe is characterized not by gender but theme. Its association with women is an empirical observation, and it is primarily through women's voices that I trace its development. But this association is not absolute, and the contrasts between male and female voices are presented here to highlight a distinction between two modes of thought and to focus on a problem of interpretation rather than to represent a generalization about either sex.
>
> In presenting excerpts from this work, I report research in progress whose aim is to provide, in the field of human development, a clearer representation of women's development which will enable psychologists and others to follow its course and understand some of the apparent puzzles it presents, especially those that pertain to women's identity formation and their moral development in adolescence and adulthood (Gilligan 1982, pp. 2, 3).

Notice the apparent inconsistency of aims in these two self-reflections, given that Gilligan's interpretations are illustrated with her research findings.

> These findings were gathered at a particular moment in history, the sample was small, and the women were not selected to represent a larger population. These constraints preclude the possibility of generalization and leave to further research the task of sorting out the different variables of culture, time, occasion, and gender. Additional longitudinal studies of women's moral judgments are needed in order to refine and validate the sequence described (p. 126).

Gilligan's research and account of care levels or care development to which the last citation refers is characterized by gender rather than theme.

Chapters three and four of Gilligan's book, which encompass care levels, refer only to Gilligan's abortion study. This study sampled women only in order to discover how women in particular think about moral issues, construct moral categories, and define moral language. Quite understandably then, Gilligan faults Kohlberg's all-male sampling because he was not researching *male* development, but supposedly, human development.

> To derive developmental criteria from the language of women's moral discourse, it is necessary first to see whether women's construction of the moral domain relies on a language different from that of men and one that deserves equal credence in the definition of development. This in turn requires finding places where women have the power to choose and thus are willing to speak in their own voice (p. 70).

Moreover, Gilligan's interpretive analysis of findings from this study focuses on gender difference by organizing the various caring themes of self-survival, feminine virtue and conformity, moral nihilism, and shared (caring) responsibility together under gender.

Yet, in addition, Gilligan characterizes her chosen moral issue, as in the abortion study, as focusing on problems of passivity and dependence that have been "most problematic for women" and as requiring a resolution of the conflict between sexist conventions of femininity and women's conception of adulthood (pp. 69, 71). The subject of the study was designed to focus on "how women deal with such choices," "bring(ing) to the core of feminine apprehension . . . that sense of living one's deepest life underwater" (p. 71).

There is not only a clear emphasis here on gender, then, but a head-on confrontation with sexism. Moreover, this confrontation occurs in an especially sexist context, a sexist crisis. While Gilligan makes the crisis nature of the abortions' study clear (pp. 72, 107), she does not make clear how much the crisis is one of sexism itself. However, Gilligan emphasizes from the start the role of sexism in women's spontaneous and distinctive moral judgment more generally. Care orientation is introduced with illustrations from female respondents which show "a sense of vulnerability" that impedes these women from taking a (moral) stand, what George Eliot regards as the girl's "susceptibility" to adverse judgments by others, which stems from her lack of power and consequent inability "to do something in the world" (p. 66). As Gilligan puts this point: "When women feel excluded from direct participation in society, they see themselves as subject to a consensus or judgment made and enforced by the men on whose protection and support they depend and by whose names they are known" (p. 67). Gilligan illustrates her point vividly, through a respondent.

As a woman, I feel I never understood that I was a person, that I could make decisions and I had a right to make decisions. I always felt that that belonged to my
father or my husband in some way, or church, which was always represented by a
male clergyman. They were the three men in my life: father, husband, and
clergyman, and they had much more to say about what I should or shouldn't do.
They were really authority figures which I accepted. It only lately has occurred to me
that I never even rebelled against it, and my girls are much more conscious of this,
not in the militant sense, but just in the recognizing sense . . . I still let things happen
to me rather than make them happen . . . (p. 67).

Again, characterizing women's moral judgment *as a whole*, Gilligan noted
that,

The essence of moral decision is the exercise of choice and the willingness to accept
responsibility for that choice. To the extent that women perceive themselves as having no choice, they correspondingly excuse themselves from the responsibility that
decision entails. Childlike in the vulnerability of their dependence and consequent
fear of abandonment, they claim to wish only to please, but in return for their
goodness they expect to be loved and cared for. This, then, is an "altruism" always
at risk, for it presupposes an innocence constantly in danger of being compromised
by an awareness of the trade-off that has been made (p. 67).

More significant, then, is a continuing emphasis on the sexism problem
throughout Gilligan's discussion and her excerpts from respondents. This
continuing emphasis is found even when Gilligan's deliberate emphasis is
elsewhere. When Gilligan and her respondents speak of relationships, over
two chapters, there is scarce mention of the relational network of siblings
and friends that supposedly define care's relational orientation. One would
expect some emphasis on a close female friend or two in an open-ended interview about one's abortion decision. While there are some abstract
generalizations about caring for "others," or for a "future child," in this
text, the only actual ongoing relationships emphasized are with "the
boyfriend" or "lover." Moreover, the egregiously sexist nature of these
relationships and of women's situations in them (especially regarding abortion) are emphasized in each case.

In discussing level 1 of care, for example, Gilligan notes that as a general
phenomenon, "Relationships are for the most part disappointing" (p. 75).
A respondent illustrates this point, "The only thing you are ever going to
get out of going with a guy is to get hurt" (p. 75). Gilligan then notes that
"as a result, women sometimes choose isolation to protect themselves
against hurt" (p. 75). Yet whether women choose isolation or not, the
overall orientation of self-care at level 1 is self-protective, not merely self-
concerned (pp. 75-77). And what women are protecting themselves against

primarily, in the responses that Gilligan cites, are the threats posed by characteristically sexist rejection in love relationships, and in social responses to the abortion crisis.

Gilligan's respondent Betty, for example, had her first abortion after being raped. Afterwards she felt "helpless and powerless to obtain contraception for herself because she did not have any money and she believed she needed her parents' permission; she also felt powerless to deal with her boyfriend's continuing harassment. In the end, she gave in to his assurance that he knew what he was doing and would not get her pregnant, influenced by her belief that if she refused, he would break up with her" (p. 109). She became pregnant again because "no one was willing to help." "After I went to bed with him he just wanted me to do everything he wanted to do . . . (disregarding) the fact that I wanted my freedom." Thus Betty becomes preoccupied with her own needs, as Gilligan puts it, "to ensure her own survival in a world perceived as exploitative."

At care level 1, a woman's thinking "focuses on taking care of herself because she feels all alone. The issue is survival." Gilligan continues, "In this mode of understanding, the self . . . is constrained by lack of power that stems from feeling disconnected" (p. 75). It is notable that Kohlberg's stages also trace an egoistic "concern for self" at his level 1 (stages one and two). However, this egoism simply expresses self-interest, not protection against hurt and threat, especially not hurt or threat that puts one's very survival at stake. Presumably this is because Kohlberg and other moral developmentalists are trying to tap general competence in responding to the broad spectrum of moral problems, not to especially oppressive or threatening ones. However, adolescents and adults are observed to retreat to this egoistic level functionally, when faced with oppressive crises and threats (as in a prison environment). In this regard it is important to note in the above citations (and those following) how often the self-protective response of self-concern at level 1 seems to follow, not precede, the level 2 concern with "maintaining one's love relationship." It is important to note how often this concern sets care up for its fall. (This ordering of concerns, by levels, is not what we would expect in a developmental sequence.)

We see this regressive "retreat from care," from hurt in love relationships, in the reaction of moral nihilism and confusion which is the corollary to self-protection in Gilligan's account.

Lisa, a fifteen year old, believing in her boyfriend's love, acceded to his wish "not to murder his child." But after she decided not to abort the child, he left her and "thus ruined my life. . . . " "I don't know what to do with my boyfriend gone. I'm still in love with him, no matter what he has done, and that really confuses me, because I don't know why I still do. . . . " "I can't get him out of my mind" (pp. 123-124).

We see a similar reaction in a woman already working out of such reactions near the highest level of care.

Sarah [a third respondent] had discovered the first pregnancy after her lover left her, and she terminated it by an abortion which she experienced as a purging expression of her anger at having been rejected. Remembering the abortion only as a relief she nevertheless describes that time in her life as one in which she "hit rock bottom." Having hoped to "take control of my life" she instead resumed the relationship when the man reappeared. Two years later, having again "left my diaphragm in the drawer," she became pregnant. Although initially ecstatic at the news, her elation dissipated when her lover told her that he would leave her if she chose to have the child (pp. 90-91).

Level 2 care is said to show a general concern for serving others' needs sacrificially and thereby winning their approval. It tries to go along with shared norms and values which define the expectations others have of you. In this respect, it seems akin to Kohlberg's conventional stage three in which respondents play their "good boy/good girl" roles as others expect of them. Gilligan faults Kohlberg's system for classifying women's judgment at such a childlike level of care (p. 70).

However, in the excerpts Gilligan cites from respondents, the orientation of level 2 is tailored much more to serving "the boyfriend's" needs and sexist expectations in particular. A secondary focus is on living up to peculiarly sexist conventions of love relations, marriage, and family. There is an emphasis here, as we saw above, on "trying to please" out of the "vulnerability of dependence" and "fear of abandonment," and in the "expectation of being loved or cared for." The prescribed manner of pleasing invokes peculiar "feminine stereotypes" such as "deference to male judgment and strength," and "gentleness and tact" (pp. 69, 79, 80). None of these key features of Gilligan's "altruism at risk" are key to Kohlberg's "good girl" orientation at conventional stage three.

Consider the types of conventionality care espouses. Gilligan notes that respondents in her abortion study got pregnant in hopes of "making the baby an ally in the search for male support and protection or, that failing, a companion in male rejection" (p. 72). Pregnancy was also seen as "the perfect chance to get married and leave home" to overcome a sense of "powerlessness and disconnection" (p. 75) or as a way "to concretize our relationship" (p. 88) or "put the relationship to the ultimate test of commitment" (pp. 72, 119). Yet abortion also was seen as a way to overcome this sense of powerlessness, to "continue the relationship [with the lover]" and not "drive us apart." "Since I met him he has been my life. I do everything for him, my life sort of revolves around him" (p. 81).

Gilligan observes that her respondent Ellen "considered herself 'fairly strong-willed, fairly in control' . . . until she became involved in an intense love affair . . . entertain[ing] vague ideas that some day I would like a child to concretize our relationship. Abjuring, with her lover, the use of contraceptives . . . she saw herself as relinquishing control, becoming instead 'just simply vague and allowing events to just carry me along' " (pp. 87-88). Even in evolving out of level 2, as Gilligan sees it, a woman "struggles to free herself from the powerlessness of her own dependence" when "pregnant by the same man" who made her have the abortion that kept them together (p. 81).

Aside from relationality, which defines the caring perspective overall, "not hurting" is its dominant orientation. Yet when Gilligan introduces this "common thread" in her initial excerpts from women's judgment, the thread that particularizes these concerns is "not hurting *boyfriends*." As one respondent puts it, "Not hurting others is important in my private morals. Years ago I would have jumped out of the window not to hurt my boyfriend. That was pathological. Even today, though, I want approval and love. . . . " As another respondent put it, "My main principle is not hurting people . . . I'm afraid I'm heading for some big crisis with my boyfriend someday, and someone will get hurt, and he'll get more hurt than I will" (p. 65).

SOCIALIZATION AND REFLECTION

The above citations and the way they are cast, I believe, are representative of Gilligan's first two levels of care. Yet Gilligan's depiction of level 2 care also includes a more general "caring for others" emphasis alongside the focus on "serving males." In recent writings (Gilligan 1987; Gilligan and Wiggins 1987) an emphasis has been placed on caring in mother/daughter relations. These emphases in care could challenge the hypothesis that care coping is tailored to sexism. However, I believe that the discussions of care and mothering are highly speculative rather than merely interpretive or qualitative in a social scientific sense. They concern a global "care orientation" that is very difficult to tie to care *levels* and to the actual interview data from which they derive. This is why I have relied so heavily on Gilligan's original, book-length account of care in these discussions. And, of course, the "care as liberation" hypothesis does not claim that care *only* involves coping with sexism.

Moreover, the emphasis on care in general, at level 2, is precisely what we should expect if care truly, as Gilligan claims, is conventional at this level. The key is that care fits traditional sexist socialization here, socialization in "service orientation" or service ideology, or a coping strategy based on this theme. Obviously the effectiveness of such a socialized conventional ideology depends on its somehow rationalizing the subservient role of women relative to men in society. And there is little dispute, I take it, that this socialized ideology does so in part by generalizing women's service orientation to others as a whole. Gilligan acknowledges this tendency by citing the Broverman, Broverman, Clarkson, Rosenkrantz, and Vogel (1970) stereotypes of gentleness, tact, and other care-taking traits as "female stereotypes" (p. 79). These socially approved and fostered traits are to characterize woman's character, her moral self-concept and orientation to others generally, in sexist society. As Gilligan also notes, this very same rationalization, viewing oneself and one's activities as *generally* altruistic, is used explicitly by women at level 2. Here it handles inner conflicts with the slavishness of conventional care. These are signs of care's strategic and partially reflective quality at level 2, as well as its more dominant socialization influence.

Therefore, if sufficient reason can be offered for preferring a socialization and reflection explanation for care over a cognitive-developmental account, the "care as liberation" hypothesis is supported. This will be our final task regarding the first two levels of care and, eventually, the third level. Since level 3 is more complex, it will have to be addressed at more levels. Since it is a primarily "self-chosen" orientation, rather than a conventional one, we will emphasize the contrast between its reflective, "consciousness-raising" character, and the nature of cognitive-developmental processes. This approach will be clarified briefly at the outset.

While level 3 care copes with sexism in particular, it also retains the generalized focus on "caring for others" begun at level 2. The "care as liberation" hypothesis holds three factors responsible for this trend. First, there is the lingering influence of conventional care at this level. This is shown by the continuation of a basic service theme from level 1, now applied to oneself as well as others, combined with the failure to notice key deficiencies of this theme during reflection. Second, there is the "slave morality" phenomenon, providing a more elaborate version of level 2 rationalizing. It "legitimizes" caring service by generalizing its apparent virtues ideologically.[3] Third, there is the influence of truly liberated "consciousness-raising" or insightful reflection. In this process, some women uncover many of the morally valid and virtuous components of benevolence as Gilligan recounts. These components properly express benevolence toward others in general. However, on the "care as liberation" hypothesis, Gilligan's account of level 3 overrates the fullness and adequacy of these discoveries. It also overates their cognitive developmental form.

To support the role of these three factors at level 3, our analysis should identify six features of care here: (1) the significant role of sexist socialization influences; (2) the superior role of reflection; (3) the peculiarly personal, insightful, or otherwise nongeneralizable form of that reflection; (4) its social-ideological character; (5) its moral defects, and the defective way that it is personalized and legitimized; and (6) the relative lack of evidence for cognitive-developmental processes there, or their significant influence. Since Gilligan cites very few level 3 respondents, it is difficult to draw extensive support for these features from the text. However, these features all receive some support in the citations that follow, especially when considered in the context of Gilligan's research approach. The moral defects of mature care, suggested earlier, are elaborated in detail elsewhere (Puka 1988). The contrast I will outline between Gilligan's research and the approach of cognitive-developmentalists she criticizes is elaborated elsewhere as well (Puka forthcoming).

The task of our analysis is made easier by the fact that socialization, reflection, and cognitive-developmental processes exert very different degrees of influences on us. As shown in the research literature, and by common observation, socialization plays the dominant role in shaping our motivations, values, and ideologies. On this same basis we can assume that the power of female socialization in sexist "service orientation" is great. Gender studies, as a field, have greatly bolstered that assumption. Reflective learning and insight are a powerful factor in forming moral ideologies among adults, where the effects of earlier socialization are weakened or overcome. (The work of Perry [1970] provides excellent evidence for this which Gilligan countenances greatly in defining level 3. This evidence is supported, despite appearances to the contrary, by Belenky, Clinchy, Goldberger and Tarule [1986] in *Women's Way of Knowing*.) The power of reflection here is greatly increased, we commonly observe, when compounded with the social reinforcements of one's reflective peers. In these contexts, the burden of proof is on the moral developmentalists (*any* moral developmentalist) to show that the processes she posits exist at all, and can compete with these others for influence.

Importantly, cognitive-developmental processes arise in the same form across the broad range of social interactions. They operate and evolve by inherent "principles" of cognitive construction, such as integration and differentiation. They form a holistic system for organizing moral experiences and affording basic but general competence in facilitating moral judgment. Such cognitive-moral processes will use experience and learn from it. Perhaps they also will encompass some reflective processes at the highest developmental levels. But they will not be determined by the peculiar shape of one's experience and socialization or the particular styles and discoveries of personal insight. Thus, for example, coming to believe in one's subservient roles and traits as a woman is not something we would expect to evolve in this way. This ideology is too particularized, too dependent on particular interpretations of fact and value and on partisan social interests to arise without being taught or "discovered" by intellect. This ideology is also regressive, presumably, rather than developmental. In the same way, coming to adopt a distinctively feminist perspective or liberal ideology is not likely to be natural and basic to women's cognitive development.

Thus to support the dominant roles of socialization and reflective coping in care, we will merely note their robust role in Gilligan's account and in her research. At the same time, we will cite the weakness of her grounds for conceiving care as cognitive-moral development. Let us begin with the reflective peculiarities of level 3, the ways care rests on certain reflective insights into particular sorts of experience, and into oneself.

Raising Consciousness

Gilligan first characterizes the transition to level 3 care in the responses of Sarah. Here Gilligan aims to show "how closely her transformed moral understanding is tied to changing self-concept" (p. 92). When asked to "describe yourself to yourself," Sarah answers quite self-consciously,

I have been thinking about that a lot lately, and it comes up different than what my usual subconscious perception of myself is. Usually paying off some sort of debt, going around serving people who are not really worthy of my attention, because somewhere in life I think I got the impression that my needs are really secondary to other people's and that if I feel, if I make any demands on other people to fulfill my needs, I'd feel guilty for it and submerge my own in favor of other people's, which later backfires on me, and I feel a great deal of resentment for other people that I am doing things for, which causes friction and the eventual deterioration of the relationship. And I start all over again. How would I describe myself to myself? Pretty frustrated and a lot angrier than I admit, a lot more aggressive than I admit (pp. 92-93).

Notice that the process of actual self-reflection (and even the awareness of that process) figures into what Gilligan sees as transformation in Sarah's level of care. As Sarah also notes, "I am suddenly beginning to think . . . the things that I believe and the kind of person I am are not so bad . . . I am a lot more worthwhile than my past actions have led other people to believe . . . you realize that that is a very usual way for people to live—doing what you want to do because you feel your wants and your needs are important" (pp. 93-94). At earlier levels, women could self-reflect when asked, but they do not report actually doing so "a lot lately."

Notice also that this process of self-reflection uncovers socialization into an explicitly sexist "service orientation," into "going around serving

people," as a respondent puts it (p. 92). "Somewhere in life I think I got the
impression that my needs are really secondary to other people's." "I am
beginning to think that all these virtues aren't really getting me anywhere"
(p. 93). It also uncovers the "cycle of repetition" and "psychology of
passivity" rationalized previously—"And I start all over again." Sarah's
usual subconscious perception of herself did not reveal these psychological
phenomena.[4]

Sarah's explicit process of consciousness-raising regarding her approach
to sexist relationships is especially clear in the following passages from
Gilligan:

For Sarah, facing a second abortion, the first step in taking control is to end the relationship in which she has considered herself "reduced to a nonentity," but to do so
in a responsible way. Recognizing hurt as the inevitable concomitant of rejection,
she strives to minimize that hurt by dealing with her lover's needs "as best I can
without compromising my own. That's a big point for me, because the thing in my
life to this point has always been compromising, and I am not willing to do that
anymore" (p. 95).

As Gilligan concludes from this case, in Chapter 3, "Thus, release from the
intimidation of inequality finally allows women to express a judgment that
had previously been withheld. What women then enunciate is not a new
morality, but a morality disentangled from the constraints that formerly
confused its perception and impeded its articulation" (p. 95).

Yet later, picking up the case again, Gilligan notes that in becoming "tired of
always bowing to other people's standards," Sarah "draws on the Quaker
tradition" in which "your first duty is to your inner voice." " . . . when the inner voice replaces outer ones as the arbiter of moral truth, it frees her from the
coercion of others (p. 118). As Gilligan continues,

Reiterating with more confidence and clarity her *discovery* of an *inner voice*, she says
that her decisions previously "were based elsewhere, I'm not really sure
where. . . . " The integration of this *insight* into Sarah's life, the completion of the
transition precipitated by the crisis, entailed a *long and painful process* that lasted
for most of the year. Through this experience, she became more *reflective*: "I see the
way I am and watch the way I make choices, the things I do." And she is now committed to building her life on a "strong foundation" of *"surprisingly old wisdoms"*
with respect to her work and her relationships (p. 122).

Again, I underline those aspects of Gilligan's citations that seem most
distinctively reflective, insightful, and peculiar to Sarah's consciousness-
raising experience. The "inner voice" of Quakerism is perhaps the most
vivid example. Note again that Gilligan does not attempt to distinguish the

peculiarly cognitive-developmental quality of these remarks. Sarah moves on to level 3 once she starts "watching herself," and "listening" to the "inner voice" she has "discovered after a long and painful process in which she became more reflective." These sorts of responses are offered by Gilligan's other level 3 respondents as well, such as Diane: (See also the case of Ruth [p. 102].)

It is part of a self-critical view, part of saying, "How am I spending my time and in what sense am I working?"

When I am dealing with moral issues, I am sort of saying to myself constantly, "Are you taking care of all the things that you think are important, and in what ways are you wasting yourself and wasting those issues?"

The only way I know is to try to be as awake as possible, to try to know the range of what you feel, to try to consider all that's involved, to be as aware as you can be of what's going on, as conscious as you can of where you're walking (p. 99).

Gilligan shows how heavily level 3 care relies on reflection by stressing the contextualism of level 3 thought. Gilligan gauges this contextualism through Perry's (1970) levels of intellectual judgment. In the transition to level 3, Gilligan tells us, women start breaking down their absolute equations between selfish and bad, altruistic and good, and start making judgments relative to situational contexts. They tentatively seek out the shades of the moral gray in moral reality, as they perceive it (pp. 102-104, 166). At level 3, this contextualism reaches fruition.

Perry's (1970) levels of intellectual development arose primarily from the reflective struggle of college students to deal with conflicts between the theories and belief systems they were exposed to in class. They chart reflective or meta-cognitive orientations and the way they change. These are orientations to our beliefs, values, and ethical systems themselves, rather than to moral problems and social interactions. When Gilligan asks women for self-descriptions relative to moral choice and receives the sort of responses cited above, she is getting at such meta-cognition. The same is true when she asks respondents to define morality itself and elicits responses such as "trying to uncover a right path to live, and always in my mind is that the world is full of real and recognizable trouble, and is heading for some kind of doom" (p. 99).

By contrast, classic moral development approaches focus on first-order questions of what to do about this or that problem. They encompass only those reflective processes which we can assume will evolve inherently in anyone, as a normal part of trying to deal with socio-moral problems in a minimally competent way. For the most part, reflective processes (and their insights) seem determined by particular types of education, exposure to ideologies and culture-specific styles of thinking, as well as the luck of discovery. At level 3, as noted, these processes are intermixed.

Social Learning and Moral Ideology

To distinguish the phenomenon of moral development from socialization and personal experience, researchers have evolved a variety of empirical and interpretive methods. Their research interviews feature a standard variety of moral dilemmas accompanied by challenging probe questions. Together these are designed to assure the existence of stable cognitive systems underlying the gamut of moral beliefs and ideologies, and expressed in them. By testing the limits of moral competence, these research probes uncover the stability of these systems, including their resistance to strong situational pulls from the environment on the one hand, and also their capacity to address varied moral situations consistently on the other. Such cognitive competence would differ from the *particular skills or beliefs we show in performing* particular kinds of tasks. Cognitive systems which show such general competence and stability, which take a holistic organizational form, are unlikely to be determined by the varying schedules of situational reinforcement. These include reflective self-reinforcement. Yet moral ideologies and skills, by contrast, seem to arise primarily in this way.

Cognitive developmental researchers also measure the transformation of cognitive systems at regular intervals to chart the mechanisms of change. In this way, they can better distinguish inherently constructional processes from shaping due to socialization, personal experience, or reflection.

By contrast, Gilligan's research uncovered care using open-ended interviews. Here respondents emitted only those dilemmas they found personally salient. Alternatively, a single, real-life dilemma was used, such as abortion. This approach does not focus on general moral competence.[5] Rather than challenging care responses to see if stable cognitive systems lay beneath, Gilligan's interviews "follow(s) the language and logic of the person's thought," only "asking questions in order to clarify the meaning of particular responses" (p. 2). This may very well have clarified moral ideology or socialization rather than cognitive-moral competence.

Gilligan's largest study ($N = 144$) was cross-sectional. It did not chart the evolution of care longitudinally at regular intervals. Her other two studies ($N = 25$, $N = 21$) involved only a single follow-up interview (pp. 2-3). On this basis, Gilligan gained little empirical sense of what prompted change in care when change occurred. Gilligan never actually observed women go through the levels of care in order or otherwise, as noted. But even more important, her writings do not illustrate the holistic structure or functioning of care levels in any *one* respondent. Rather Gilligan reconstructs the care sequence of development *conceptually* in her book, by glimpsing a small interval of development in eight respondents (p. 108). Care at each level, and as a general orientation, is presented as a reconstructed composite of responses across respondents.

Furthermore, Gilligan's abortion study, so key to defining care levels, pulled for unusual responses. As noted, it utilized a dilemma which all involved considered a desperate personal crisis for respondents (p. 108). In fact, Gilligan's developmental analysis of these responses was termed "magnification of crisis." This indicates Gilligan's stated belief that care development is a form of "response to crisis" in particular (p. 107). As Gilligan sees it, we will move up care levels only if we have sufficient self-confidence and sense of control over our lives when facing crisis. Where we meet rejection and hurt with vulnerability and despair, we will likely regress (p. 76-78, 123-126). It is unclear how much these psychological states or processes involve cognitive systems at all, much less morally competent and self-constructional ones. In any event, these sorts of processes are highly vulnerable to socialization influences and peculiarities of personal experience. Gilligan does not try to distinguish aspects of cognition that succumb to this vulnerability from those which do not. This is especially problematic in the abortion context where ideological positions on this issue are so prominent in social experience.

On the contrary, "No claims are made about the origins of the differences described" in Gilligan's account, differences in moral theme or self/other perspective or gender. Rather, the account acknowledges the shaping influence on care of social status and power, traditional gender stereotypes, sexual politics, and bad experiences in love relationships. Feelings of loneliness and depression play a role too (pp. 2-3).

Finally, Gilligan reports great changes in care during a mere one-year interval. Out of 21 respondents in the abortion study, eight developed and four "got worse" between pre-test and post-test (p. 108). Such a degree of change is unheard of where the inherent, constructional processes of cognitive development are at work (e.g., integration, differentiation, equilibration). Yet while change of this sort would be expected in moral ideology or reflective beliefs, especially during personal crises, Gilligan never poses such interpretations of her results. She also does not try to distinguish functionally regressive change in care performance from regression in the cognitive-developmental organization of care competence.

Against these observations of socialization and personal reflection in care stand Gilligan's few remarks on how women "construct" care levels, on how one level is a more "differentiated and comprehensive" transformation of the level before (pp. 73, 76, 78). These are key cognitive-developmental catchwords. The "care as liberation" hypothesis acknowledges that Gilligan may have uncovered some strands of cognitive structure in care. However, there is no indication in her account that these strands are sizable or that existing theories of development cannot encompass them under other moral themes. Gilligan's remarks are so sparse, when seen in relation to any standard cognitive-developmental account (Walker 1984), that they are best viewed as suggesting a different sort of account. Otherwise, they bear serious deficiencies.[6]

Conclusion

"Care as liberation" is meant to be a working hypothesis. Its degree of support is to be compared with Gilligan's "different voice" interpretation of what her observation indicates. In providing this support, I have attempted to illustrate care's primary concern with women confronting sexism, and the primary role of socialization, personal reflection, and coping involved. I hope it is obvious how much this discussion and the "care as liberation" hypothesis extend the feminist potential of care, and of Gilligan's voice.

NOTES

1. Gilligan's sweeping criticisms of Piaget, Erikson, and especially Kohlberg have reduced the credibility of care unnecessarily (Gilligan 1982, pp. 12-22, 31, 45, 59, 66, 99, 104; Kohlberg 1984, pp. 338-370; Broughton 1983).

2. The hypothesis borrows explicitly from "radical therapy" notions of "abstraction" and "personalization" in the ideological rationalization process. Some observers may find them questionable. However, these powerful notions might also have been derived from Gilligan's own consideration of how "abstraction" and "impersonality" enter patriarchal morality. Likewise the slave morality or "resentment" phenomenon can be identified in ideologically neutral terms.

3. Again, while some women learn the lessons of sexist abuse at levels 1 and 2 and face the inadequacies of their coping strategies and rationalizations, they mistakenly personalize responsibility for failure. As they evolve a more balanced and selective approach to care coping, they rationalize its lingering limitations through the ideology of selective generalization and equalization of (slavish) care. Thus, care at level 3 still constitutes service orientation, service to others generally, but now not to the extent that oneself is left out.

4. I believe we would term these realizations especially insightful—psychological and interpersonally insightful—and recognize that they are tailored to the issue of sexism primarily. We should not expect "the average woman" across cultures to come up with such distinctive ways of thinking simply because she takes a relational perspective and is therefore concerned with not hurting others.

5. Gilligan used Kohlberg dilemmas in some studies, but primarily for purposes of comparing justice reasoning with the alternative care orientation her interviews

uncovered. Gilligan criticized Kohlberg's dilemmas and probe questions for discriminating against care orientation (Gilligan 1982, p. 100; Gilligan and Belenky 1980).

6. Since Gilligan did not observe development over a significant length of time in these studies, she could only conceptualize how each level of care *might* have been constructed from another, not how they actually appeared to be. Such a constructional analysis might easily be provided of any two conceptually related ideologies, one of which is more sophisticated than the other. In addition, Gilligan does not actually explicate the difference between levels and transitions, showing how the latter stabilize into holistic equilibrated systems. She does not actually trace each key component of care from one level to the next, showing how it is transformed and reintegrated with each other (and with new cognitive differentiations) to form a functioning whole. Even the three defining features of care—its moral theme of helping and not hurting, its relational perspective, and its notions of responsibility to others—are not depicted at all three levels. Level 1 seems to lack all of them. The remaining two-level sequences might just as well be conceived as a bi-modal phenomenon, rather than a developmental sequence. Finally, key features of care that distinguish each level pop in or out of the care "sequence" without clearly being transformed, differentiated, or reintegrated in cognitive organization. Among these are, (1) "survival orientation," which disappears at level 3, (2) the "concern for good," of level 2, which is later *replaced* by the "concern for truth," and (3) the need to be "honest with oneself" in level 2 to 3 transition which does not appear to evolve from, or evolve into, any concern like it. The greatest deficiencies in Gilligan's account, however, were noted earlier. Gilligan's approach to research and interpretation simply does not provide for crucial distinctions between socialization, consciousness-raising, and cognitive development.

REFERENCES

Belenky, M., Clinchy, B., Goldberger, N., and Tarule, J. (1986). *Women's ways of knowing*. NY: Basic Books

Bettleheim, B. (1943). Individual and mass behavior in extreme situations. *Journal of Abnormal and Social Psychology 38*:417-452.

Broughton, J. (1983). Men's virtues, women's rationality. *Social Research 3*:597-642.

Broverman, I. K., Broverman, D. M., Clarkson, F. E., Rosenkrantz, P. S., and Vogel, S. R. (1970). Sex-role stereotypes and clinical judgments of mental health. *Journal of Consulting Psychology 34*:1-7.

Chodorow, N. (1978). *The reproduction of mothering: Psychoanalysis and the sociology of gender*. Berkeley: University of California Press.

Freud, A. (1946). *The ego mechanisms of defense*. NY: International University Press.

Gilligan, C. (1986). Exit-voice/dilemmas in adolescent development. In *Development, democracy, and the art of tresspassing*, ed. A. Foxley, M. McPherson, and G. O'Donnell. Indiana: University of Notre Dame Press.

————— . (1982). *In a different voice: Psychological theory and women's development*. Cambridge, MA: Harvard University Press.

————— . (1986). Reply by Carol Gilligan. *Signs: Journal of Women in Culture and Society 11*:324-333.

Gilligan, C., and Belenky, M. (1980). A naturalistic study of abortion decisions. In *New Directions for Child Development*, ed. R. Selman and R. Yando. San Francisco: Jossey-Bass.

Gilligan, C., and Wiggins, G. (1987). The origins of morality in early childhood relations. In *The emergence of morality in young children*, ed. J. Kagan and S. Lamb. Chicago: Chicago University Press.

Jennings, W., and Kohlberg, L. (1983). Effects of just community programs on the moral level and institutional perceptions of youthful offenders. *Journal of Moral Education 12*:33-50.

Jennings, W., Kilkenny, R., and Kohlberg, L. (1983). Moral development theory and practice for youthful and adult offenders. In *Personality theory, moral development, and criminal behavior*, ed. W. Laufer and J. Day. Lexington, MA:Lexington Books.

Johnston, K. (1985). *Two moral orientations—two problem-solving strategies: Adolescents' solutions to dilemmas in fables*. Ed.D. diss., Harvard Graduate School of Education.

Kohlberg, L. (1984). *The psychology of moral development*. NY: Harper and Row.

Kohlberg, L., Kauffman, K., and Scharf, P. (1975). *Corrections manual*. Cambridge, MA: Moral Education Research Foundation.

Langdale, C. (1983). *Moral observations and moral development*. Ed.D. diss., Harvard University Graduate School of Education.

Lyons, N. (1983). Two perspectives: On self, relationships and morality. *Harvard Educational Review 53*:125-143.

Miller, J. B. (1976). *Toward a new psychology of women*. Boston: Beacon Press.

Nicholson, L. (1983). Women, morality and history. *Social Research 50*, (3):514-536.

Noddings, N. (1984). *Caring*. Berkeley, CA: University of California Press.

Perry, W. (1970). *Forms of intellectual and ethical development in the college years*. NY: Holt, Rinehart and Winston.

Puka, B. (Forthcoming). Justice and care, Kohlberg and Gilligan: In many different voices. *Human Development* (journal).

————— . (1988). Ethical caring: Pros, cons and possibilities. In *Inquiry into values*, ed. S. Lee. NY:Mellen Press.

Sanford, N. (1955). The dynamics of identification. *Psychological Review 62*:106-118.

Walker, L. (1984). Sex differences in the development of moral reasoning: A critical review. *Child Development 55*:677-691.

3

Sometimes I Feel Like a Motherless Child: The Call and Response for a Liberational Ethic of Care by Black Feminists

Toinette M. Eugene

The social situation of the black extended family in these remaining decades of the twentieth century evokes from many black individuals and from the core of many typical black communities the lament of the black spiritual, "Sometimes I feel like a motherless child." This melodiously mournful lament is more than a mere commentary on the individual desolation and disorganization that accompanied the shock of enslavement a "long way from home." Expressed as both a call and response, it also intentionally conveys the loss of West African political, religious, and family systems which attached great importance to the public role of mothers as well as fathers within the traditional black community. This lament of the motherless child reflects an historical reality of the Afro-American community—all have shared in the oppressive experience of being deprived at some time of a mother's attention because of the inordinate demands of a racist society competing for possession of her person.

Slaves came from social systems in their African homelands in which men and women shared power and were economically independent. Slaves and their posterity correctly perceived their new life in the United States as "a war on African familyhood— . . . those expressions and manifestations of individual/community/national life and organization which emerge from the African world view of relationships between Man, Woman, and the Universe" (Carruthers 1979, pp. 3–9). The slaves not only lost their homeland, they also lost a social system whose culture and social organization were guided by the obligation and the ethic of care for kin. The policies grew out of a liberational ethic.

In this chapter I shall reflect on aspects of this Afro-American ethic of care as liberation which is regularly practiced and embodied by black women. I do not suggest this ethic involves and identifies burdened representatives of what is pejoratively understood as "women's work." Rather it is evidenced in the lives of those mothers and moral agents of the race whose self-initiated expressions of care have undergirded the survival of a people. They have indeed secured a future legacy that is humane, holistic, and compassionate for all who choose to belong to their unfolding and liberating extended families.

I will argue that black women are not special specimens of womanhood; rather, they are women who have been given less protected and more burdensome positions in society. As Michele Wallace (1979) has so poignantly pointed out, this has resulted in the "myth of the superwoman," which is not a description of black women but, rather, a measure of the difference between what is regularly expected of white women and what is essentially required of black women.

Within this understanding, I will note the distinguishing characteristics evident in the activity of black women which move them beyond some limiting levels of care-giving. These limitations of care-giving are consistent with or similar to some white women's social and personal condition of subordination to the service of men and children (Frye 1983). Within this understanding I will presume for black women as Nel Noddings (1984) presupposes for white women, a particular moral agent, one who is clear about the boundaries of the self so that she can practice the demanding tasks of engagement without the fear of accompanying loss of self. This acceptance of the potential "loss of self" is not understood by most black women as the inevitable experiential result of the effects of sexism and racism, but rather is claimed as an acceptable risk of willingly participating in the religious and Christian paradox of following in the example of Jesus. Consequently, deriving from this evangelical understanding, an Afro-American ethic of care as liberation also requires attention to issues of justice as well as to issues of care, concern, and connection.

Finally, I do concur with the compelling reflections of Bill Puka's (this volume) hypothesis on "care as liberation," although my sociohistorical overview goes beyond his summary remarks dealing with "slave morality and other ideologies."

MOTHERHOOD AS A MANIFESTATION OF CARE AND AUTHORITY

Aspects of the black religious and political experience in the United States reflect elements of this ethic of care and "familyhood" as attested to uniquely by black women. In both sacred and secular community settings, there are powerful and respected older women who are addressed by the title, "Mother" (Carter 1976). This title is meant to be a tribute to generativity more than to the biological reproductivity of black women. It is the self-initiated and communitywide respected vocation of those who are called "Mother" to care for those in need and to make a way where there is no way—a way of justice, a way of equity, a way that may serve as a highway of righteousness for everyone who wants to walk with integrity. These terms which define the work and role of motherhood for the motherless are cast intentionally in the biblical and religious context which is endemic to black experience in this country. The relationship of black women to religion for the sake of forging a liberational ethic of caring will be reviewed at length later in this chapter.

In secular settings, such mothers are often the heads of black women's organizations and hold positions of power and authority in more broadly based community and civil rights organizations. In sacred places, particularly within the churches, they are occasionally pastors, sometimes evangelists, more often pastors' wives and widows, but most often leaders of organized church women (missionaries, deaconesses, mothers' boards, etc.). Regardless of their institutional offices, these women wield considerable authority in both sacred and secular settings. The members of the community call them "Mother" and their "children" are often religious and political leaders who owe their power and authority to the sponsorship of such respected and revered women.

At present, sociopolitical as well as theological movements dominated by white feminists are forcing rapid reorganization of traditional expectations based on gender. Black women's absence from or their reluctant or ambivalent participation in these white feminist movements is overwhelmingly evident (Gilkes 1979; Hemons 1980; Noble 1978). Although black women evince a clear understanding of their multifaceted exploitation by white Americans, male and female, they are ambivalent about aiming the same criticism at black institutions and black men (Hoover 1979; Wilson 1980). The complicated response of black women to the women's liberation movement represents an implicit understanding that black women's roles and status within the black community are qualitatively distinct although not independent from their roles and status within the dominant society. Black women, at various levels of consciousness, know that many of the feminist theories and critiques of American society simply do not fit the facts of their experience.

Since much of the work involved in social change, group survival, and community politics takes place at the local level, black women's church and community leadership is important and valued. Black women's church work generally encompasses active membership in local churches, clubs, and religious auxiliaries, as well as teaching Sunday school. Addressing such women as "Mother" signifies the community's recognition of the importance of their various roles and length of service in the public institutions of Afro-American community life.

Women who are addressed and referred to as "Mother" within the context and by members of the Afro-American community are those whose influential power, biblical righteousness, and personal authority embody the epitome of the liberational ethic of care alive and active within the group. The needs of those who experience the vicissitudes of life as motherless children are thus attended to in a fashion that the dominant white society would never affirm or in most instances acknowledge as legitimate or valuable.

CHURCH AND COMMUNITY MOTHERS AS ETHICAL CARE GIVERS

The roles of church and community mothers represent impositions of Afro-American familistic and pseudofamilistic ties upon social organization and the process of social influence. These mothers serve effectively for a very long time and accumulate great prestige and in many cases very real institutional authority. Not only are they venerable role models, and power brokers, but the actuarial realities of black life are such that elderly black women provide the continuity necessary to promote unity in the face of ever changing historial conditions. Such women are the senior members of diverse networks of community workers and provide a counterforce to the potential for fragmentation.

In some religious settings, these women provided continuity through the crises wrought by the deaths of charismatic local and national leaders. Their particular organizational roles and degree of power vary from one organization to another. Still their roles as "Mother's" are part of a larger tradition of female leadership and care-giving at various levels of community life. Finally, these mothers, bridges between the women's world and the world of men, exercise authority not only in the autonomously organized world of black women but also in areas dominated by black men.

A SOCIOECONOMIC BACKDROP FOR THE ETHICAL CONTEXT OF BLACK WOMEN

Nonetheless, the combined force of the inherited oppressive experiences of race, sex, and economic discrimination impose on the vast majority of black women a severely disadvantaged status. In response to these dynamics, black women in their development, analysis, and appraisal of various coping mechanisms against the white-oriented, male-structured society do not appeal to fixed rules of absolute principles of what is right or wrong, or good or bad. Instead, they embrace alternative values and a liberational ethic of care related to the causal conditions of their cultural circumstances.

The cherished assumptions of dominant ethical systems predicated upon both the existence of freedom and a wide range of choice have proven false in the real, lived, black life. Thus, black women have created and cultivated a set of ethical values that allow them to prevail against the odds, with moral integrity, in their ongoing perforce participation in the white male-capitalist value system.

The moral situation of black women in contemporary society is still a situation of struggle, a struggle to survive collectively against the continuing harsh historical realities and pervasive adversities in today's world. The determining existential circumstance in which black women find themselves in the 1980s is little better than the situation was in the 1880s. Federal government programs, civil rights movements, and voter education programs have all had a positive impact on black women's moral situation. They have not been able, however, to offset the negative effects of the inherent inequities which are inextricably tied to the history and ideological hegemony of racism, sexism, and class privilege (Cherry et al. 1962; Clarke 1971; Davis 1982; Deutrich and Purdy 1980; Hull, Scott, and Smith 1982; Jackson 1975; Jones 1986; Ladner 1971; Lerner 1972; Rose 1980; Steady, 1981).

The persistent obstacles of poverty, gender discrimination, and racial prejudice continue to enslave black women and their families to hunger, disease, and the highest rate of unemployment since World War II (Facts 1985). Education, housing, health care, and other necessities which were gained during the mid and late 1960s are deteriorating faster now than ever before. The National Urban League (1987) in its publication, *The State of Black America 1987*, provides the supporting data of how the significant formal institutions in American life—the government, the national economy, and education—functionally divert options of equality for black women in general and for black female heads of families in particular (National Urban League 1987).

Afro-American women find that their situation over the past 100 years has constructively changed only for a few and has worsened for many. In dispelling some of the myths about the benefits that black women have reaped from the new economic and political order of the American society, Sylvia Parker writes in "Negro Women's Progress,"

Statistics on pay and job level always can be tailored to mislead, if not to lie. That's one of the first lessons a serious reporter of economics-like-it-is must learn. I've just relearned it in a new Census Bureau study tracing the progress of Negro women since 1960.

The figures seem to show that the Negro woman, for decades at the very bottom of the U.S. economic ladder, is finally moving rapidly ahead and that she is even pulling ahead of the Negro man (Wright 1969, p. 50).

She concludes; "In sum, from next to nothing to a little may be a giant statistical step. But in real life, it's a baby's crawl" (Wright 1969; see also Gump 1979; Puryear 1980). According to the latest contemporary demographic studies on census and salary ranges for various sex and race groups, black women still earn the least.

Abbey Lincoln demythologizes black women's social progress in her cryptic depiction of the contemporary black woman by describing why she often "feels like a motherless child":

Her head is more regularly beaten than any other woman's, and by her own man; she's the scapegoat for Mr. Charlie; she is forced to stark realism and chided if caught dreaming; her aspirations for her and hers are, for family's sake, stunted; her physical image has been criminally maligned, assaulted, and negated; she is the first to be called ugly, and never beautiful. . . . (Lincoln 1966, p. 18).

This is the socioeconomic backdrop for the call and response for a liberational ethic of care by black women. The context by which black women's moral situation is understood and assessed consists of

all those women who toiled under the lash for their masters, worked for and protected their families, fought against slavery, and who were beaten and raped but never subdued. It was those women who passed on to their nominally free female descendants a legacy of hard work, perseverance, and self-reliance, a legacy of tenacity, resistance, and insistence in sexual equality—in short a legacy spelling out standards for a new womanhood (Davis 1981, p. 29).

The values that black women have derived for themselves and have offered as options to the black community as well as to the members of a broader, dominant society cannot be understood or adequately explained apart from this historical context in which black women have found themselves as moral agents and ethical care givers. Moreover, the liberational ethic of care which black women have provided and modeled as a legacy to the black community, as well as to the feminist movement in U. S. society, is rooted in a distinctive religious consciousness and in deliberate religious traditions which have been irrepressible in redeeming and transforming an entire human environment.

A selective overview of black religious history reveals that value indicators of public activism coupled with evidence of self-sacrificial personal endurance are emblematic of the liberational ethics of care expressed by black women. It is historically documentable that whenever black women have lived out these value indicators, they have proved to be liberational for both the Afro-American population and for other diverse feminist communities.

Social activism, self-sacrifice, and other similar value indicators of a liberating black ethic of care may be verified in the lives of Mother Mary McLeod Bethune and Nannie Helen Burroughs, to name but two exemplary models. However, these value measures and these valuable models of a black liberational ethic of care represent more than unusual courage and strength; they also represent realistic responses to economic deprivation and political and social inequality. Most black women have been forced to perform labor and to take risks that few white women have been called upon to do either in the name of religious traditions or on behalf of the survival of their race.

It is obvious that black women have experienced oppressive structures of racism, class bias, and male supremacy in both religion and society in this country. What is not always so obvious to a dominant white world-view and even to feminist theological understandings is that Afro-American culture and religion have generated alternative inter-related notions of womanhood different from those of mainstream American economics, society, and theology (Eugene 1984). These alternative experiences, visions, and images of womanhood have been forged out of the furnace of a moral value system endemic to the black church. The following text will explore, through an interpretation of black religious traditions in which black women share, aspects of the moral consciousness and value system of liberational caregiving that guides black women in their ongoing struggle for survival.

BLACK WOMEN AND MORAL VALUES DURING SLAVERY

Historically, the Black Christian Church has been the fiery furnace through which systematic faith affirmations and liberating principles for biblical interpretation have been developed by Afro-American people. Within this "invisible institution," hidden from the observation of slave masters, black women, along with black men developed an extensive moral value system and religious life of their own. In the language of moral development theorist, Carol Gilligan, (1982) they established and operated out of a "web or network of relationships" and intimacy with others in community. The moral values of care, compassion, and cooperation with other black and oppressed persons served as criteria for decisions and actions intended to lay hold of the good, the true, and the beautiful. The particular moral leadership of black mothers who were not afraid to risk the loss of self for the sake of the family was a dominant factor in sustaining the life and hope of the Afro-American community struggling to emerge out of slavery into what they described biblically as the freedom of the children of God. This particular expression of moral leadership is thus clearly expanded beyond Gilligan (1982) and Noddings's (1984) theories and qualities of an ethic of care.

The biblical interpretations of the antebellum Black Church which provided black people with webs of relationships centering on the God of justice and of liberation made slaves incontestably discontent with their servile condition. The moral value system of black people in this period encouraged slave women, whose bodies and spirits were wantonly violated by the immoral sexual advances of white masters, to eliminate the sources of their oppression in order to maintain and sustain their fragile nexus with God, community, and self as valued and trusted friends. Paula Giddings, in her text *When and Where I Enter: The Impact of Black Women on Race and Sex in America* (1984), reports on the moral resistance black slave women offered:

So, by the early eighteenth century an incredible social, legal, racial structure was put in place. Women were firmly stratified in the roles that Plato envisioned. Blacks were chattel, White men could impregnate a Black woman with impunity, and she alone could give birth to a slave. Blacks constituted a permanent labor force and metaphor that were perpetuated through the Black woman's womb. And all of this was done within the context of the Church, the operating laws of capitalism, and the psychological needs of White males. Subsequent history would be a variation on the same theme.

In its infancy slavery was particularly harsh. Physical abuse, dismemberment, and torture were common. . . . Partly as a result, in the eighteenth century, slave masters did not underestimate the will of their slaves to rebel, even their female slaves. . . . But Black women used every means available to resist slavery—as men did—and if caught, they were punished just as harshly (Giddings 1984, p. 39).

In the midst of this dehumanizing slave environment, black families survived. They overcame the slaveholders' attempts to reduce them to so many subhuman labor units, managing to create an ongoing system of family arrangements and kin networks. Domestic life became critically important, for it was the only place where slaves had any equality and autonomy as human beings (Gutman 1976).

Regarding domestic life and labor, Angela Davis (1981), in *Women, Race, and Class* has observed a paradox of great significance for black women and men:

The salient theme emerging from domestic life in the slave quarters is one of sexual equality. The labor that slaves performed for their own sake and not for the aggrandizement of their masters was carried out on terms of equality. Within the confines of their family and community life, therefore, Black people managed to accomplish a magnificent feat. They transformed that negative equality which emanated from the equal oppression they suffered as slaves into a positive quality: the egalitarianism characterizing their social relations (Davis 1981, p. 18).

Mother Harriet Tubman, as she was known to the community and countless others, provided egalitarian images of slave women as strong, self-reliant, proud of their roots and of their ability to survive, convinced of their right to a place in society through the liberation of all black people. Equally oppressed as laborers, equal to their men in the domestic sphere, they were also equal in their moral resistance to slavery, participating in work stoppages and revolts, fleeing north and helping others to flee.

At a women's rights convention in Akron, Ohio in 1851, several of the most celebrated examples of early black feminist ethics of care as liberation were rendered by the legendary abolitionist and mystic Sojourner Truth in her famous "Ain't I a Woman" speech. From the very beginning of the conference, the white women were overwhelmed by the jeering ridicule of men who had come to disrupt the meeting. Their most effective antagonist was a clergyman who used both the gender of Jesus and the helplessness of the women to counter their feminist arguments. Sojourner squelched the heckler by correcting his theology first, noting that Jesus came from "God and a woman—man had nothing to do with Him" (Davis 1981, p. 236). Second, Truth asserted that women were not inherently weak and helpless.

Raising herself to her full height of six feet, flexing a muscled arm, and bellowing with a voice one observer likened to the apocalyptic thunders, Mother Truth informed the audience that she could outwork, outeat, and outlast any man. Then she challenged: "Ain't I a Woman?" (Davis 1981, p. 235). She spoke of women's strength and moral abilities to set things aright: "If the first woman God ever made was strong enough to turn the world upside down all alone, these women together ought to be able to turn it back, and get it right side up again. And now they are asking to do it, the men better let them" (Davis 1981, p. 236). Clearly the liberational ethics of caregiving asserted by black women who give credence to the black Judeo-Christian tradition honor reconciliation as highly as liberation. Although I disagree with Mother Truth's theology concerning the origin of sin and disorganization in the world, I do believe that the liberational ethic of care which goes beyond the barriers of race is paradigmatic and distinctive in the consciousness of black women. The accumulated experiences and expressions of black women during slavery were nuanced and nurtured by their webs of relationship with the Black Church and its biblical interpretations of the salvific power of God.

EMANCIPATION, MIGRATION, AND MORAL EDUCATION FOR BLACK WOMEN

The institution of chattel slavery in the United States was destroyed by the most momentous national event of the nineteenth century, the Civil

War. Emancipation removed the legal and political slave status from approximately four million black people in the United States. This meant that, in principle, these blacks owned their persons and their labor for the first time. Unfortunately for the vast majority of Afro-Americans, the traditional practices of racial and gender subordination continued to subject them to incredible suffering after that war.

Black women began a life of freedom with no vote, no constitutional protection, and no equity. Black women, young and old, were basically on their own with no political or educational structures of support or affirmation. The patterns of exploitation of the black woman as laborer and breeder were only shaken by the Civil War; by no means were they destroyed. Throughout the late nineteenth and early twentieth centuries, black women were severely restricted to the most unskilled, poorly paid, menial work. Virtually no black woman held a job beyond that of a domestic servant or field hand. Keeping house for white patrons, sharecrop farming, and rearing children for white families continued to dominate all aspects of the black woman's life.

The systematic oppression and routinized exclusion of black females from other areas of employment confirmed the continuation of the servile status of black women. As Jeanne Noble describes it, "While freedom brought new opportunities for black men, for most women it augmented old problems" (Noble 1978, p. 63). After emancipation, racism and male supremacy continued to intersect patriarchal and capitalist structures in definitive ways.

The religious consciousness of the black freedwoman in the latter nineteenth century focused of necessity on elevating the black community. The black female was taught that her education was meant not only to uplift her but also to prepare her for a life of service in the overall community. In the religious understanding and moral consciousness of the black community this life of service and care-giving was not to be that of the "domestic mule." Rather, her role was that of servant-leadership which was authoritative in its exercise of stewardship in behalf of the community or family. The religious consciousness and caring attitude of black women as servant leaders in the best sense is very similar to Nel Noddings, that there is "a readiness to bestow and spend oneself and make oneself available" (Noddings 1984, p. 19).

However, this ethic of care enacted and articulated by black women is not in any way to be construed as a "slave morality and mentality," although it may be rendered so from a white perspective. The liberational ethic of care articulated and expressed by black women is in fact a reaffirmation of Carol Gilligan's final stage in care orientation when women realize that "responsiveness to self and responsiveness to others are connected rather than opposed" (Gilligan 1982, p. 61).

There was a general attitude regarding practical education and formative ethical preparation for black feminists, says historian Jeanne Noble, that "Negro women should be trained to teach in order to uplift the masses" (Giddings 1984, p. 101). This attitude provided an additional impetus for black women, such as Nannie Helen Burroughs, Charlotte Hawkins Brown, and Mother McLeod Bethune to found schools. Although the curriculums of these schools included academic subjects, there were large doses of industrial arts courses, and an environment that fostered strict codes of social and sexual morality as well as a praxis of economic ecology. Consumerism was never included or encouraged in the curricular offerings explicitly emphasizing value clarification for black young women. Within the context of these lyceums of moral and survival education, it was biblical faith grounded in the prophetic tradition that helped black women to learn strategies and tactics designed to make black people less susceptible to the indignities and proscriptions of an oppressive white social order.

During the mass migration of southern blacks to the North (1910–25) tens of thousands of black women and men left home, seeking social democracy and economic opportunity. During this colossal movement of black people, the Black Church continued to serve as the focal point and center for maintaining the moral value system and the network of relationships which sustained community life.

Not surprisingly, this accelerated movement of blacks out of the South had a direct economic impact on black women's lives. Black women migrated North in greater numbers than black men. Economic necessity dictated that most black women who immigrated to urban centers find work immediately. Struggling to survive themselves and to provide for their families, black women once again found only drudge work available to them.

Simultaneously while the black woman was trying to organize family life according to black traditional roles, the white male-dominated industrial society required that she serve as a catalyst in their labor transition process. Her own unfamiliarities and adaptation difficulties had to be repressed. She was responsible for making a home in crowded substandard housing, finding inner-city schools that propagated literacy for black children, and contributing with other relatives to provide enough income for her family to cover the most elementary needs of survival and sustenance.

The moral and religious value system of the Black Church served as a sustaining force and as an interpretive principle that guided migrant black women in facing life squarely, in acknowledging its raw coarseness. The white elitist attributes of thoughtless passivity and an enervative delicacy, considered normative for femininity were not functional in the pragmatic survival of black women. Cultivating conventional amenities was not a luxury afforded them. Instead, black women were aware that their very lives depended upon their being able to decipher the various sounds in the larger world, to hold in check the nightmare figures of terror, to fight for basic freedoms against the sadistic law enforcement agencies in their communities, to resist the temptation to capitulate to the demands of the status quo, to find meaning in the most despotic circumstances, and to create something where nothing existed before. The expression of a liberational ethic of care for black women meant and required a "sheroic" self-sacrifice and self-giving that could not ever afford public displays of feminine softness, shyness, silence, or diffidence as a response indicating servile subservience.

From the period of black urban migration through World Wars I and II, black women who were rooted in the strong moral values and prophetic traditions of the Black Church became national crusaders for justice. Mother McLeod Bethune and her associates recorded and talked about the grimness of struggle among the least visible people in the society. Bethune, adamant about the unheralded achievements of black women, encouraged them to "go to the front and take our rightful place; fight our battles and claim our victories" (Smith 1980, p. 152). She believed in black woman's "possibilities," moral values, and their place on this earth.

In response to the hostile environment, deteriorating conditions, and the enduring humiliation of the social ostracism experienced by black people especially during these war years, Bethune and company exposed the most serious and unyielding problem of the twentieth century—the single most determining factor of black existence in America—the question of color. In their strategic attacks against the ideological supremacy of racist practices and values, they appealed to the religious traditions of black people that began in their invisible church during slavery.

CONTEMPORARY BLACK FEMINIST CONSCIOUSNESS AND AN ETHIC OF CARE

The ability of black people to cope in a hostile society has endured into the twentieth century; studies of black women in urban situations show that the means by which black families survived slavery still enable black women and their families to survive today (Malveaux 1985; Smith 1985; Burnham 1985; Facts, 1985; Higginbotham 1984).

Within this historical framework of past and present hostility, black women have always perceived networks of relationality in the liberation struggle differently from white women; domesticity has never been seen as entirely oppressive but rather as a vehicle for building family life under slavery; male/female relationships have always been more egalitarian; there has more often been less emphasis on women's work as different from and inferior to men's; slaves and freed persons, male and female, have consistently tended to rebel against the sexual oppression of black women as well as the emasculation of black men.

It is easy to understand why many black people today see the white feminist movement as an attempt to divide black people along gender lines and issues (Joseph and Lewis 1981). Many contemporary black feminists caution against espousing more "radical" white feminist stances because they regularly leave out, as irrelevant, black men, black children, black families. A primary moral value of black people is articulated in the overarching and enduring black feminist position: solidarity among black women and black men is essential for survival.

Given that this primary moral value of solidarity among blacks and with other people of color and with other oppressed communities of resistance is a sine qua non, an argument can be made that such a liberational ethic of care could provide an alternative perspective for the feminist movement as a means of greater unification. All oppressions stemming from domination and subordination are connected, and as such, this black feminist ethic of care based on this kind of solidarity could offer a method of liberation and reconciliation that may at least lessen stratification based solely on gender, class, and color.

A dramatic statement of black women's unique attitude toward solidarity with black men is found in the 1977 statement of the Combahee River Collective, a black lesbian feminist group from Boston.

Although we are feminists and lesbians we feel solidarity with progressive Black men and do not advocate the fractionalization that white women who are separatists demand. Our situation as Black people necessitates that we have solidarity around the fact of race. . . . We struggle together with Black men against racism, while we also struggle with Black men about sexism (Combahee River Collective 1981, p. 213).

These black lesbian feminists explicitly rejected a feminist separatism that equates all oppression with sexual oppression and that fails fully to comprehend the reality that black women *and* men are victims of shared racial oppression. Feminist separatism is not a viable political philosophy for most black women. Ethicist Barbara Hilkert Andolsen, in her remarkable assessment of racism and American feminism, *Daughters of Jefferson, Daughters of Bootblacks* (1986), issues a strong caveat to white women who want to understand the black feminist experience:

Those of us who are white feminists need to be careful that we do not articulate limited strategies for dealing with sexism as if they were the only legitimate feminist strategies. White feminist separatist theories or strategies that ignore the strong bond forged between many black women and men in a shared struggle against racism do not speak to all women's experience (Andolsen 1986, p. 98).

White feminists who seek to enjoy a relationship of "sisterhood" or at least that of solidarity for the sake of coalition-building with black women, have a responsibility to learn about black women's perspectives on feminist issues, to analyze how racist social structures may distort the impact of white feminist proposals, and to support black women in their self-defined struggle for liberation. Black feminists are creating their own analyses of sexism and of the interconnections between racism and sexism. White feminists who are seeking to contribute to an inclusive feminist cosmology that respects and reflects the diversity of women's experience need to learn from the experiences, moral values, and feminist philosophy articulated by black women.

Moreover, both black and white feminist groups that do not give explicit attention to the realities yoking racism and sexism will find that they can be easily manipulated by dominant males who appeal to unexamined class and race interests to achieve economic exploitation of all women. Work and dialogue between feminists of color and white feminists in this essential area is, in some sense, just beginning.

Both in informal day-to-day life and in the formal organizations and institutions of society, black women are still the victims of the aggravated inequities of the tridimensional phenomenon of race/class/gender oppression. It is in this context that the moral values of black women and the emergence of black feminist consciousness shaped by black biblical and religious traditions must continue to make a decisive difference for a debilitated and nearly dysfunctional human environment.

BLACK RELIGIOUS TRADITIONS AND WOMANIST MORAL VALUES

Because of the religious traditions from which most black women have come, the Bible is most often regarded as the highest source of authority in developing and delivering a black moral praxis and an ethic of liberational care. By selectively utilizing the content of the prophetic authors in the Hebrew Scriptures, black women have refuted the stereotypes that have depicted black people as ignorant minstrels or vindictive militants. Remembering and retelling the Jesus stories contained in the Scripture of the early Christian community has helped black women to deal with the overwhelming difficulties of overworked and widowed mothers, of underemployed and anxious fathers, of sexually exploited and anguished daughters, of prodigal sons, and of dead or dying brothers whose networks of relationships are severely weakened or threatened. The call and response for a liberational ethic of care for the motherless and needy is ever present in the dynamics of any black community of faith and action. The leadership of black women who bear and wear the title of Mother within that religious and civic community is paradigmatic and exemplary of the transformation of power that the ethic contains.

Black feminist consciousness and mothering moral values grow out of and expand upon black, biblical hermeneutics in order to reweave what has been ripped asunder in the black family and community by racism, sexism, classism, and capitalism. The prophetic tradition of the Bible and the Black Church have empowered black women to fashion a liberational ethic of care on their own terms. This ethic heals and transforms, as well as destroys the negative orientations that stem from the bankrupt values of the larger and politically dominant society. Also, the feminist truths and moral values espoused by contemporary black women articulate possibilities for decisions and actions which address forthrightly the circumstances that inescapably shape black life.

Flowing from black women's biblical faith grounded in the prophetic tradition, many black women have been inspired to hold in high regard a diaconal model of black feminist theology which is consistent with their experience and identity. Without rejecting all white feminist models of theology that focus on mutuality and equality as sine qua nons of liberation, many black feminists choose a theology of servant leadership which has been espoused by Christ Jesus. This biblical model of feminist liberation theology is principally focused on human solidarity with those who suffer or who are marginalized in any way. A much greater examination, integration, and expression of this black feminist ethical perspective and alternative to "mainstream" models of feminist ethics of care is needed (Eugene 1984).

A theology and praxis of servant leadership abides within black feminist consciousness, or black *womanist* consciousness, to use Alice Walker's concept. In the introduction to *In Search of Our Mothers' Gardens* (Walker 1983), Walker proposes several descriptions of the term "womanist," indicating that the word refers primarily to a black feminist and is derived from "womanish," that is, outrageous, audacious, courageous, or willful behavior (Walker 1983, pp. xi–xii). To be a faithful womanist, then, or to operate out of this system of black ethical care-giving which flows from biblical understandings based on justice and love, is to express in word and deed an alternative ontology or way of living in the world that is endemic to many black women. It is precisely black womanist religious responses of endurance, resistance, and resiliency offered in the face of all attempts at personal and institutional domination that may provide a renewed ethical legacy of liberation for everyone concerned.

Walker adds that a black womanist is "committed to survival and wholeness of entire people, male *and* female. Not a separatist . . . traditionally universalist . . . traditionally capable . . . " (Walker 1983, p. xi). The practical implications of such meanings for interaction and dialogue between black women's moral values and the diverse tenets of white feminist ethics are obvious and challenging.

In exploring the implications contained in Walker's richly descriptive prose, it is possible to make some concluding reflections on a black liberational ethic of care and on the contribution of black women's life experiences and mothering activity as they interface with white feminist perspectives.

Black womanist responses formulating a liberational ethic of care are meant to be alternative standards of womanhood, contradictory and paradoxical to those of mainstream white American society. Black womanist responses articulating a liberational ethic of care for those who experience themselves to be orphaned, abandoned, alienated, and marginalized are meant to be paradigmatic of an entire and authentic religious community of the oppressed. A liberational ethic of care embraces not only the implications and results contained in the New Testament narratives of the passion, death, and resurrection of Jesus Christ, but is also a referent for the related prophetic, liberating tribulations through which so many other oppressed suffering servant-leaders such as Mother Sojourner Truth, Mother Harriet Tubman, Mother Jarena Lee, Mother Amanda Berry Smith, and Mother Mahalia Jackson have come also. Womanist moral values are expressed through radical healing and empowering actions with those who are considered as the very least in the Reign of God and also in the harsh reality of this present secular world.

Black womanist ethics of liberational care expressed as an "appreciation for the struggle, a love of the folk, and a love of self—*regardless*" (Walker 1983, p. xi), encourage a continual and open means of interaction between those who claim diverse womanist and feminist identities and experiences. Black womanist ethics of liberational care mitigate against the oppression of all who are literally or symbolically motherless children.

Black womanist ethics of liberational care insure action on behalf of justice as a constitutive element in the nurturance of those who are without any other viable means of support, concern, or protection. To heed the call and to respond by exercising this ethic of care for the orphans and alien of our society means "to take care of business" instead of doing business "as usual." The status quo structures of the social order are intended to be shaken and shifted by those designated as Mothers and invested with authority and leadership on behalf of those in need. Those who are able to recognize this distinctive role and responsibility as it emanates out of the Afro-American community, and who utilize a methodology of personal risk for the sake of transformational results in society, are most welcome to participate and to extend a long-standing ethical tradition of efficacious care.

REFERENCES

Andolsen, B. H. (1986). *Daughters of Jefferson, daughters of bootblacks: Racism and American feminism*. Macon, GA: Mercer University Press.

Burnham, L. (1985). Has poverty been feminized in black America? *The Black Scholar*, March–April, 14–24.

Carruthers, I. (1979). War on African familyhood. In *Sturdy black bridges: Visions of black women in literature*, eds. P. Bell, B. J. Parker, and B. Guy-Sheftall. Garden City, NY: Doubleday-Anchor.

Carter, H. A. (1976). *The prayer tradition of black people*. Valley Forge, PA: Judson Press.

Cherry, G., Thomas, R., and Willis, P. (1962). *Portraits in color: The lives of colorful Negro women*. Paterson, NJ: Pageant Books.

Clark, H. H. (1971). The black woman: A figure in world history. *Essence*, June, 36–44.

Combahee River Collective (1981). A black feminist statement. In *This bridge called my back: Writing by radical women of color*, eds. C. Moraga and G. Anzaldua. Watertown, MA: Persephone Press.

Davis, A. Y. (1981). *Women, race, and class*. New York: Random House.

Davis, M. W. (1982). *Contributions of black women to America*. New York: Urban League.

Deutrich, M. E. and Purdy, V. C., eds. (1980). *Clio was a woman: Studies in the history of American women*. Washington: Howard University Press.

Eugene, T. M. (1984). Black women contribute strong alternate images. *National Catholic Reporter*, April, 13, 4.

Facts on U.S. Working Woman. (1985). *Black women in the labor force*. U.S. Department of Labor, Women's Bureau, Fact Sheet No. 85-6, July.

Frye, M. (1983). *The politics of reality: Essays in feminist theory*. Trumansburg, NY: The Crossing Press.

Giddings, P. (1984). *When and where I enter: The impact of black women on race and sex in America*. Toronto: Bantam Books.

Gilkes, C. T. (1979). Black woman's work as deviance: The sources of racial antagonism within contemporary feminism. (Working Papers in Progress, No. 66). Wellesley, MA: Wellesley College, The Stone Center.

Gilligan, C. (1982). *In a different voice: Psychological theory and women's development*. Cambridge, MA: Harvard University Press.

Gump, J. (1979). Reality and myth: Employment and sex role ideology in black women. In *Psychology of women: New directions for research*, eds. J. Sherman and F. Denmark. New York: Psychological Dimensions.

Gutman, H. (1976). *The black family in slavery and freedom, 1750–1925*. New York: Pantheon Books.

Hemons, W. M. (1980). The women's liberation movement: Understanding the black woman's attitude. In *The black woman*, ed. L. Rodgers-Rose. Beverly Hills, CA: Sage Publications.

Higginbotham, E. (1984). *Employment for professional black women in the twentieth century*. Memphis: Memphis State University Research Clearinghouse.

Hoover, T. (1979). Black women and the churches. Triple jeopardy. In *Black theology: A documentary history, 1966–79*, eds. G. Wilmore and J. Cone. Maryknoll, NY: Orbis Books.

Hull, G. T., Scott, P. B. and Smith, B., eds. (1982). *All the women are white, all the blacks are men, but some of us are brave*. Old Westbury, NY: Feminist Press.

Jackson, J. (1975). A critique of Lerner's work on black women. *Journal of Social and Behavioral Sciences, 21,* 63–89.

Jones, J. (1986). *Labor of love, labor of sorrow: Black women, work, and the family from slavery to the present*. New York: Vintage Books.

Joseph, G. and Lewis, J. eds., (1981). *Common differences: Conflicts in black and white feminist perspectives*. Garden City, NY: Anchor Press/Doubleday.

Ladner, J. (1971). *Tomorrow's tomorrow: The black woman*. Garden City, NY: Doubleday and Company.

Lerner, G. (1972). *Black women in white America: A documentary history*. New York: Random House.

Lincoln, A. (1966). Who will revere the black woman? *Negro Digest*, September, 18.

Malveaux, J. (1985). Current economic trends and black feminist consciousness. *The Black Scholar*, March–April, 26–31.

National Urban League (1987). *The state of black America 1987*. New York: National Urban League.

Noble, J. L. (1978). *Beautiful also are the souls of my black sisters: A history of the black woman in America*. Englewood Cliffs, NJ: Prentice Hall.

Noddings, N. (1984). *Caring: A feminine approach to ethics and moral education*. Berkeley, CA: University of California Press.

Puryear, R. (1980). The black woman: Liberated or oppressed? In *Comparative perspectives of third world women: The impact of race, sex, and class*, ed. B. Lindsey. New York: Praeger Publishers.

Rose, L. R. (1980). *The black woman*. Beverly Hills, CA: Sage Publications.

Smith, B. (1985). Some home truths on the contemporary black feminist movement. *The Black Scholar* March–April, 4–13.

Smith, E. M. (1980). Mary McLeod Bethune and the National Youth Administration. In *Clio was a woman: Studies in the history of American women*, eds. E. Deutrich and C. Purdy. Washington DC: Howard University Press.

Steady, F. C. (1981). *The black woman cross culturally*. Boston: Schenkman Publishing Company.

Walker, A. (1983). *In search of our mother's gardens: Womanist prose*. San Diego: Harcourt, Brace, Jovanovich.

Wallace, M. (1979). *Black macho and the myth of the superwoman*. New York: Dial Press.

Wilson, G. (1980). The self-help actualization of black women. In *The Black Woman*, ed. L. Rodgers–Rose. Beverly Hills, CA: Sage Publications.

Wright, N. (1969). Black power vs. black genocide. *The Black Scholar, 1,* 50.

4

Pragmatism, Feminism, and Sensitivity to Context

Charlene Haddock Seigfried

Carol Gilligan's work (1982) is usually read as making two claims of particular interest to those engaged in the area of moral development, but whose implications range far beyond any one disciplinary field. The first is the empirical claim that women and men, as a matter of fact, differ in their approaches to moral reasoning, with women emphasizing care and men justice. The second is the value claim that since an ethics of care is at least equal to, and perhaps better than, an ethics based on fairness, moral theory—which has traditionally emphasized justice and ignored or trivialized caring relationships—ought to be restructured to take account of the importance of caring. The first claim is problematic in ways that the second is not. In exploring some of the different assumptions underlying the two claims and some of the consequences of acting on them I will be drawing on a reconstructed pragmatism to suggest an alternative approach to the first and a defense and expansion of the second.

I have serious reservations about the value of research which reinforces the stereotypical association of "care" with women and "justice" with men, rather than investigating the constellation of factors which have given rise to this stereotype and its impact on women's and men's gender identities and social situations. Therefore, I will seek to show how associating these orientations with situations primarily and gender only secondarily will lead to more worthwhile results than continued empirical research intended to demonstrate that women's moral reasoning differs in kind from men's. This is not an attempt to impose moral standards on an otherwise neutral scientific methodology but to point out some consequences for research programs of the realization that values and expectations are always already incorporated into empirical research. On the other hand, I think that there are good reasons to support the second

claim that 'care' as a primary ethical orientation has been devalued because
of its association with women and that the dimension of care ought to be
central to any system of moral reasoning worth supporting.

IDENTIFYING DIFFERENCES OF MORAL REASONING WITH GENDER

The empirical claim has not been satisfactorily demonstrated so far, but
there is some evidence to suggest that there are aspects of moral reasoning
that show up more clearly in women's than in men's responses. Whatever
future investigations in this area may turn up, it seems to me that any differences that are found to distinguish women's and men's responses can be
better accounted for by identifying the common traits of the situations of
those for whom 'care' plays a larger role and distinguishing these from the
traits found in the experiences of those who respond in terms of 'justice'.
We now know enough about the different expectations of and behaviors
toward male and female infants and children to realize how large a role
socialization plays in the formation of one's sense of self as male or female.
We also know that human individuals are not simply imprinted, but that
from at least birth on, if not before, they actively respond to and reject such
environmental constraints in unique ways. Furthermore, clusters of traits
assigned on the basis of sex have been found to reflect the negative evaluation of women compared to a positive evaluation of men. Therefore, we do
not need a value-neutral assignment of traits that are assumed to be male or
female, but a critique of the ways in which certain personality and behavior
traits have been differentially assigned to women and men in any given
society.

Once it is realized that maleness and femaleness are mutually constructed, in
interaction between individuals and their social milieu, including their primary
caretakers, then it is as misleading to try to identify traits as specifically female
as it is to deny that similar socialization processes can produce similar 'second
natures' or patterns of behavior, including reasoning processes, in men. If
some traits, such as particular patterns of reasoning, are found dispropor-
tionately in women, then what we have discovered is a successful set of circumstances for producing that trait. But because of the variability in the circumstances of growing up I would expect to find variability in the occurrence
of the trait, that is, it will not be found in all women and it will be found in
some men as well. But because of the wide dissemination and acceptance of sex
stereotyping I would also expect to find some divergences along gender lines.
The exact distribution can only be empirically determined.

Once it is realized that the 'naturalness' of sexual identification can no
longer be maintained, then the rationale for attributing traits on the basis of

sex would have to change radically. The questions we would need to ask about any such project also change. Instead of: "What does this tell us about women?" "How would we respect this difference in deference to women's importance?" and "Why has not this undeniable difference been noticed before?" the more appropriate questions would include: "What does this tell us about the way women are brought up?" "Has the inculcation of this trait differentially in women been generally beneficial or harmful to them and to society as a whole?" and "What expectations do we as researchers bring that allows this trait to emerge and what expectations prevented it from being apparent before?"

The claim that women differ significantly from men is welcome news for those feminists who 'valorize' the feminine and argue that women's special way of being in the world has been both ignored and trivialized. But for feminists who are working for equal treatment it is seen as a misguided attempt to claim for women those very characteristics which have been traditionally attached to women and which have provided justification for treating them as inferior. It is both possible and desirable to be sensitive to both these concerns when examining Gilligan's work. Among the first questions that have been raised about her research is whether women actually do differ in the specific ways that she claims they do. The evidence is not yet all in, but most of it so far disproves Gilligan's claim of gender-related moralities, while holding open the possibility that some differences correlated with gender exist (Bebeau and Brabeck 1987; this volume).

However, this empirical question as to the existence of gender-based differences cannot be raised, researched, or resolved outside of the context of expectations, beliefs, values, and practices of those formulating the question, of those responding to it, and of those interviewed. Consequently, I do not expect that any empirical findings can determine whether women and men reason differently about moral situations just because they are women and men. This does not rule out the possibility that empirical research can validate or disconfirm the claims that most, some, or all women differ from most, some, or all men in the way they arrive at moral decisions. Even if some such findings were made, we would still have to determine to what they were attributable, that is, to make the causal connection. And this could not be decided without recourse to certain, more basic beliefs and values, such as whether one believes in biological or psychological determinism or psychosocial constructivism.

I think that specific modes of thinking and holding values arise from transactions within contexts. Thus, I would expect that insofar as women are found in similar situations that share some features that differ systematically from men's experiences, they would also share insights into the generic traits of these experiences, and develop values appropriate to such insights.[1] The more a woman's situation approximates a man's—in expectations, upbringing, opportunities, self-esteem, physical prowess, etc.—the more her and his insights and values would converge. Since gender is so strongly marked in our society, it is unlikely that women's and men's situations are ever identical, and since so much of a culture is also shared, it is also unlikely that women's and men's situations are totally different, but there would be varying degrees of sameness and difference. At one extreme, gender differences would be insignificant in comparison with other differences like talent, while at the other extreme gender differences would overwhelm and define all other differences. But most would fall somewhere in between. Bebeau and Brabeck's research (this volume) supports this expectation of similarity when women and men share similar contexts of profession and education.

I reject biological reductionism and its psychological corollaries and attribute gender differences, like all other interesting human variations, to an individually creative response, including a genetic component, to patterns of culture, socialization, and belief structures; in short, to 'nurture' interacting with 'nature' to such an extent that we can only distinguish them functionally by adopting different methodologies and having different ends in view (Seigfried 1985). Insofar as it is shown that some or most women approach ethical questions differently from some or most men, we should be interested in discovering the conditions that bring this about and the reasons why some women do not exhibit this difference. What are the positive and negative outcomes of this difference? Are the positive values being recognized by the persons holding them and by others not holding them? If it is determined that these differences allow values to be expressed that have positive significance for other persons and in other situations, then the investigation into the conditions of their development will give us a basis for determining a strategy for disseminating these values. If it is determined that the same conditions also generate values that negatively impact on those holding them or on others, then what can be done to begin to eliminate this aspect of the conditions and the values?

These preliminary questions are being raised to break down the simplistic equation of women with care and nurturance and men with justice and autonomy. It is meant to de-center the gender issue and replace it with engendering. Since to be female or male is not to instantiate an unchangeable nature but to participate in an ongoing process of negotiating cultural expectations of femininity and masculinity, then what does it mean to investigate the factual basis for the claim that women's moral reasoning is different from men's? It means at least the recognition that a specific value component is being added to, and also found to be already a part of, both the social construction of gender and its investigation. Empirical investigation does not just disclose facts of nature. For instance, insofar as it is shown that a particular configuration of values is strongly tied to women's socialization, then two outcomes are predictable. One is that this cluster of values, including processes of moral reasoning which interpret and apply them, will be found to have suffered the same trivialization and devaluing as the oppressed group with which it is associated. The proper response would seem to be the reclamation and positive revaluation of this cluster of values. The other is that these values will be found to have been inculcated in such a way as to have contributed to the subordination of the oppressed group, namely women. The proper response to this finding would seem to be to root out of the cluster and its inculcation whatever has contributed to these negative outcomes.

AN ETHICS OF CARE

The value claim that informs Gilligan's research can best be defended by calling into question major assumptions that support traditional ethical systems. I will defend the claim that there is an aspect of caring that ought to be central to value systems. The fact that women seem to realize this more than men must not be allowed to debase either the value or women. Not only women but any systematically oppressed group will experience the world differently from those not oppressed. It can be expected that there will be various degrees of assimilation to the values of the dominant group and that there will also be selective rejection of some of its values and substitution of other values and patterns of judgment. These differences are due to the dynamics of situations, including individual patterns of development, and not to women's supposed 'nature', and therefore particular values can be linked to specific interactive processes that can be investigated. Not all women experience the world identically as women, and these differences can be crucial. Likewise, patterns of oppression can be found that link sexism, racism, classism, and homophobia, which is not to deny that specific differences are also present and just as important to take account of (see Eugene, this volume).

Although the dominant group will generalize their experiences and values and dignify them as neutral, objective, and universal, they are no less partial and constrained by the conditions in which they were developed. Universalizability as a criterion of ethics or value systems should be unmasked for the drive for domination which it is. It should be replaced with a recognition of the diversity of values that have been developed to answer to different needs and a search for what is required for a harmonious community based on cooperation rather than cooptation and domination. Caring is initially a value because someone holds it to be so, but to be continuously reaffirmed as such and to be accepted by others, it must be judged by evaluating the outcomes that follow from holding it. Since these have historically been both negative and positive, the original understanding and practice of caring should be investigated and modified to bring out more strongly the beneficial aspects and to lessen the negative ones.

Women have also been oppressed through their caring and this is not entirely due to the trivialization factor. We know from personal experience as well as historical hindsight the devastating effects of assigning care to women as a means of assuring that their labor, goods, and very persons will primarily benefit men. As Beauvoir (1974 p. 288) put it: "To identify Woman with Altruism is to guarantee to man absolute rights in her devotion, it is to impose on women a categorical imperative." Some feminists have recently nonetheless linked care with women by claiming that women's nature as women so informs every aspect of their being that all women, merely by being born a woman, think, feel, act, work, and dream in gender-specific ways. This deliberate reduction of the social construction of gender to a natural process of hormones and blood can only exacerbate rather than lessen the negative effect of associating care with women, despite the best intentions of valorizing it.

I develop a model which assumes the social construction of gender, one which avoids this negative aspect by emphasizing the contextual basis for the perceived differentiation rather than the gender basis (Seigfried 1984). This does not mean ignoring the specific ways in which women express caring as central to ethics nor ignoring the consequences of the societal assumption that women must define themselves as the caring sex. This reconstruction of the empirical claim that caring is uniquely linked to women also involves showing how, given women's situation, they often need to reject or modify their care approach and develop other values like autonomy. In situations where care is eclipsed by overemphasis on other values like abstract justice, the opposite would be the case. Insofar as men are systematically socialized into over-developing autonomy and justice from a position of dominance, then these values are also necessarily distorted and have to be revalued and reconceptualized.

What has been conceptualized according to essentialist models as care versus justice and relatedness versus autonomy, thus converting "function[s] of reorganization into metaphysical realit[ies]," needs to be reconceptualized according to the pragmatist model which understands these distinctions not as "ideal objects," but as "patterns for use in the reorganization of the actual scene" (Dewey 1957, p. 51). Such distinctions as that of care versus justice are better understood as a "cooperative interaction of two distinguishable sets of conditions, so that although knowledge of them *in their distinction* is required in order that their interaction may be brought under intentional guidance," they are not isolated in practice, where "personal-social factors" intertwine (Dewey 1946, p. 321).

Much of the controversy over a "woman's morality" arises because of a misplaced faith in the possibility and desirability of an objective, neutral description of the world. Comtian positivism developed this myth of scientific neutrality just in time to infect the newly emerging science of experimental psychology with it. But the contemporary history and philosophy of science of Bas Van Fraasen, Nancy Cartwright, Stephen Toulmin, Thomas Kuhn, Paul Feyerabend, and Evelyn Fox Keller, not to mention the powerful critiques developed by their predecessors, Antoinette Brown Blackwell, William James, John Dewey, C. I. Lewis, and Friedrich Nietzsche, have thoroughly disproved this assumption of a neutral descriptivism. Every description incorporates a particular "angle of vision" and value orientation. It would be odd if women's moral development, too, as women, and by this I mean insofar as they are socialized as women and/or encounter stereotypical responses to their gender, would not bear traces of this situatedness, to the same extent that men do (Seigfried 1982). Why is it so often assumed, in formulating an ideal morality against which actual moral development is measured, that it must be one which applies universally, that is, in this case, equally to women and men, in order for it to be exemplary? Why is it assumed that if a morality develops out of some women's unique experiences, then this restricted origin, as such, would invalidate it? This is a fallacy not only of false universalism in general, but specifically of the centuries-old habit of taking the categories which men have developed from their point of view as absolute, thus covering over their one-sidedness in male experience (Beauvoir 1974, p. 290).

If it can be shown that no value claims can be universally applicable without distortion, self-deception, casuistry, or violence, then the fear that 'women's' values may not apply equally to men is irrelevant. If it can be shown that all interpretations of experience, because they are value-laden, are partial and limited, then the fact that some values are demonstrably typical of some women's situations is no criticism of them. Furthermore, if patterns of moral development and systems of ethics which claim to be both gender neutral and universally applicable, that is, human, can be shown to be, in fact, male biased and situation bound, then a hypocritically impossible task is being imposed on educational theorists to prove that their woman-centered theories can also be neutral and universal according to a pattern that disguises its own partiality.

This should not be taken as an endorsement of any particular factual claim, by Gilligan, Noddings, or others, that they have identified values which originate in women's differential development. What I have been advocating is a reconsideration of the context of investigation and discussion. The title of Gilligan's first book, *In A Different Voice* (1982), has been taken by her and others in this controversy to mean, "in a *woman's* voice." Therefore, what voice is this different from? Why, a man's voice, of course. Simone de Beauvoir's characterization of woman as "the *second* sex" in her book of that title is meant to point out that insofar as woman has been taken to be other than man she has been understood as less than him; there has been no reciprocity between men and women "for man represents both the positive and the neutral, as is indicated by the common use of *man* to designate human beings in general; whereas woman represents only the negative, defined by limiting criteria" (Beauvoir, 1974, p. xviii).

To be sure, Gilligan wants to encourage the reciprocity of men, men's interests, and men's values, with women, women's interests, and women's values. But as critics have already pointed out, this can not be done as long as women, as such, are devalued in comparison with the valued group, men. But the answer cannot be to show that women's values are not essentially theirs but are also applicable to and teachable to men, as long as the criterion of acceptability is seemingly neutral, that is, a man would also find it valuable and so claim it as a moral enhancement, but surreptitiously male/rational, that is, it is acceptable only on the terms already found to be congenial to another way of thinking, as, for example, Kohlberg's stages.

Ironically, I think it is only by de-centering the genderization of the caring-nurturant ethic that women can come out of the closet of patriarchal society and reclaim these values. Let us accept the claim that the care-nurturant ethic *is* "a different voice"—not *the* different voice, the 'other' standing in dialectical opposition to the 'same' voice, that is, the essential, the male—but one voice among many other different voices, not only of justice, but of liberation, of the greatest happiness, of *jouissance*, of the *Ubermensch*, of "growth for the sake of growth," etc. Feminists have taught us not only to distinguish between biological sex and socially constructed gender, but also between gender and individual persons. Rousseau's sexist remark that men are only men at times, but women can never forget their sex has the intention of imprisoning women in their gendered roles and freeing men to think of themselves as limiting their maleness to a few occasions and assuming an expansive humanness on most other occasions. Consequently, they can think of themselves, for instance, as making moral decisions strictly from a calculation of justice and not as a particularly male way of categorizing actions. That justice is a fundamental value may or may not be a particularly male perspective, but the consequence of simply assuming that one's assessment is neutral is to be empowered to dismiss criticisms arising from other perspectives as 'interested' and 'merely subjective.'

One reason for some women's negative response to "a woman's morality" is surely a legitimate reaction to the predictably asymmetrical pattern that results—namely, they would then be forced to choose between a "woman's morality" and "morality." Few defenders of traditional moralities have ever claimed that they were "men's moralities," despite their creation by men and obvious encoding of their interests. This not only pits "woman's morality" as a part against the whole, but also as a partial and therefore distortive view against the impartial and therefore sovereign overview.

Therefore, I would advocate a plurality of voices, which instantiate values particularized as they develop out of specific contexts and are reflectively affirmed or denied. The origin of values neither legitimizes nor delegitimizes them. Only reflective affirmation, based on the congruency of the effects of holding them with the outcomes desired, can do that (Dewey 1929). But their origins in some special angle of vision will contribute to their appeal to those similarly situated and provide the concrete basis without which discussions of morals remains aridly casuistic. There may be a recognizable set of characteristics typical of 'women's values, just as there are of 'men's' values, in societies which strongly mark gender, and these characteristics will vary independently not only among societies, but also among individual members of societies. Theories of moral development are interested in women and men, not 'woman' and 'man', and therefore care should be taken to distinguish in individual developmental sequences not only how far particular women and men converge with or diverge from societally based gender stereotypes but, more importantly, the extent to which the association of some values with women has led to their devaluation, whether found in women or men.

Not only do some women recognize their own moral development in Gilligan's account and others do not, but some men recognize themselves. Despite Freud's reductionism, not all values have their origins in our development of gender identity, but surely some of them do. Despite Marx's economic reductionism, not all values reflect economic disparities, but surely some of our values are class based. It would be much more profitable to study which developmental contexts lead to an emphasis on care and which to an emphasis on abstract principle, how one orientation or the other is fostered or discouraged, and what factors, including but not limited to gender, are part of these various contexts. The statement by Bebeau and Brabeck (this volume) that "moral sensitivity is an ability that can be developed" and their suggestions for research projects are good examples of what I mean. But we will continue to find what we expect to find in a nonproductive way that will not resolve current disputes unless we explicitly recognize and discuss the purposes that guide our findings, chief among which is the determination of what we take to be the desired moral outcome, that is, our definition of moral maturity. The factual dispute over whether moral development can be differentiated by sex cannot be profitably resolved unless we are clear about what such a finding would mean in terms of the goals we take to be most desirable.

Gender is not just socially constructed, it is also individually assumed, and its boundaries can be much looser than we care to admit. By looking at gender as a process and not as an accomplished fact, women and men are better served by learning what the effects of assuming certain values has both on their sense of their gender and on their interaction with other aspects of self and world. Because nurturance and caring have been linked to nonassertiveness and passivity as values particularly appropriate for women in certain contexts, such as those permeated by patriarchal value systems, does not establish either that they are necessarily linked together as values or that they are necessarily linked to women. Women in our society are both expected to be and are perceived as being more nurturant and less assertive than men. If nurturance is good and submissiveness is bad, it would seem desirable—and therefore reasonable—to investigate not only what the conditions are that develop such values in women, but also the relevant variants, such as which conditions generate the same combination of values in men, which generate nurturance but not submissiveness, which submissiveness but not nurturance, etc. This would enable us to understand better which antecedent conditions are more favorable for desired outcomes and therefore provide reasonable guidelines for promoting them. By asking questions in terms of desired outcomes and not just insofar as they relate to a factual determination of existing conditions, a whole new range of possibilities emerges. This way of thinking avoids some of the problems associated with uncritically identifying care with women.

It is widely acknowledged that there are not just two versions of values, his and hers, but not so widely recognized that there also are not just two gender orientations. What different cultures have selected as a suitable range of behaviors for males and females varies so widely that it is surprising that we have not been more perplexed than we seem to be in assigning such a wide array to only two types. Another way to put this is to point out that of all the ways of thinking of ourselves that of identifying ourselves as male or female as our primary orientation toward the world is much less productive of outcomes desired than any number of other orientations, for example, as creative, as free, as caretakers, as curious, as hardworking, etc. Just as we have outgrown thinking that our place in life is naturally determined by birth, so perhaps it is time to discard the belief in the natural assignment to one of two rigidly defined categories of gender. This cannot be successfully carried out, however, without first identifying and exposing the crippling effects of rigid gender assignments and rescuing those aspects of human behavior that we approve of, but which have been unfairly limited by gender.

A JUST COMMUNITY APPROACH: CONTEXTUALIST OR UNIVERSALIST?

If we link the notion of contexts which instantiate values with the understanding that each of us, singularly and as members of groups, takes in the world according to our varied perspectives, our limitations become an advantage rather than a detriment to our understanding of our relatedness within the world. Since what is apparent from one angle of vision is not necessarily available to other perspectives, we are dependent on each other's disclosures of reality. Most of us accept the scientific assumption that facts can validate or invalidate theories, but we are generally less aware of the extent to which our beliefs, expectations, and values permit or obscure the recognition of some facts rather than others. Women's unique angles of vision can therefore be affirmed, as well as the correlative need for the interaction of many such interpretations in order to compensate for the blind spots of any one.

The understanding of moral development as specifically women's or men's and as needing correction by reference to an ideally neutral and independently generated moral system of values, can thus be recognized as being both inadequate to the multitude of overlapping contexts and the cause of much unnecessary confusion in the search for Platonic values that precede and exist independent of particular human contexts. Just as we have many contexts in which persons interact, with different describable features, so there are many ways to categorize these contexts according to the ends or purposes we have in mind, for example, insofar as they further some women's or men's nurturing relations with others or insofar as they lead to a just distribution of goods, offices, and services. One way of transcending the particularity of context is to identify desired outcomes. For example, every family is unique and yet also shares some goals in common. Moral judgments grow out of reflection on experience and the codification of such findings as beneficial or not. In this way features of a morality are developed that span more than one context, but not necessarily all contexts. The convergence toward principles of wider and wider extent is a project to be achieved, subject to constant reassessment, and not a preexistent given.

Ann Higgins argues for a morality that is universal and necessary and not open to negotiation (this volume). Nel Noddings also wants to construct "a genuinely universal interpretation of culture," despite the fact that she links the companion concept of universalism, the "equity model," with the male perspective that equates humanness with maleness (this volume). Higgins enunciates a feminist position that values cannot be relative "since feminism holds equality between the sexes as a universal, nonrelative value and the elimination of social injustices due to one's gender as an absolute good." As the best means for achieving the elimination of injustice to women due to sexism she suggests the model of a just community approach to moral education. Moral growth occurs in this democratic setting through "stating an idea, listening to others agree or disagree with it, taking other's perspectives and considering their ideas, modifying one's own, restating it and listening again" (Higgins, this volume). The only check on this respect for one's own and other's opinions is that both the opinions and the way they are expressed help build a just community.

I would argue that absolute goods and universal, nonrelative values make poor bedfellows with the democratic ideal and democratic processes. These represent two largely incompatible approaches to value formation that will sooner or later collide. The ultimate norm in the community as proposed, for instance, is the justness of the community being developed. But this presupposes someone knows what a just community is. Since the students are portrayed as coming to this conclusion through the process itself and the teachers are responsible for the process being democratically fair, it is ultimately the teacher's understanding that must prevail, no matter that this is done in a noncoercive way. But the democratic process, as process, will only work if each person's perspective is genuinely respected as a contribution to the shape the community is taking. The strong peer group pressure in any such setting is toward conformity to group standards. The question then arises: whose norms? whose community? If the values and norms of the group are already set and the teachers play a game with the students to get them to work out by trial and error what these are, then the democratic process is only a facade and does not differ from group indoctrination, such as that operative in Alcoholics Anonymous meetings, where all discussion and acting-out is directed to a predetermined goal. This goal is often discussed but never itself subject to veto or modification.

In sharp contrast, in the democratic process there is no 'king', no binding arbiter, no absolute values, goals, or procedures that are not set by the group itself. What about the injunction to continue the process as process? This is an absolute value only relatively, that is, it is binding only as long as the group continues to bind itself by it. The secession of the southern states which precipitated the American Civil War is elegant testimony to the always possible move to refuse to be bound by that process. Jefferson had already clearly drawn the conclusion that if the people within the democratic process are genuinely responsible for the shape of their own political governance, then constant revolution cannot in principle be ruled out. But, as we know, in the Western democracies there is not continuous anarchy, but considerable continuity. Higgins can argue that this stems from the adherence of members of the group to certain universal moral principles, such as the oft cited Bill of Rights. But this sidesteps the issue of how these moral imperatives came about in the first place, which ones are continued and expanded, which ones quietly dropped, and what they mean concretely. On each of these issues we can trace the actual democratic process of give and take, compromise, and impassioned plea that brought and are continuing to bring them about. If absolute values played any role, they were only as tokens. Every side, and there were and are many more than two, claimed to be bound by eternal values. The only thing eternal about them is the eternal struggle to claim one's own insights as the only true understanding of them.

The power of a genuinely followed democratic process is that it starts out by recognizing that no one has a monopoly on 'eternal' values and then provides a means of developing a community that will work, despite the lack of common agreement, and without resorting to coercion. What Oliver Wendell Holmes argued, and what most nineteenth-century jurists did not want to hear, is that there is no way to interpret law in a democratic society without creating new law, new precedent. To do otherwise is to shackle people to forms of justice developed in one historical period, with all the limitations this implies. Feminists have nothing to fear from abandoning a positivist understanding of values as eternal, since as one of the groups not present when these 'eternal' values were first articulated and propagated, their well-being was not inscribed in them. The 'eternal' truth that "all men are created equal" gave way after great struggle to the 'temporal' truth that "former black slaves are created (partially) equal," and after even more struggles, to the truth—the exact moment when it became a value can be temporally located—that all women are (partially) equal. We still have not worked out what it means in practice for "all persons to be equal." The appeal to any phrase which purports to state once and for all what this means theoretically, as though this can be done in isolation from practice, is a vain appeal to a wished for certainty of a value not subject to further revision. To call any phrase the expression of an 'eternal' truth or an 'eternal' value rather than one which has been temporally determined is to devalue the creative thought, the blood, sweat, and tears which have made it, not found it to be, a value. Eternal values are supposedly self-evident and we have yet to see any such.

When, in the construction of a just community, it is determined that 'justice' includes that women participate in the same way as men in building up the community, this is not the result of appealing to a universal norm of justice. Far from it, universal justice has been thought for millennia to be compatible with women's differential participation in an ideal community. This norm is being created in its enactment, and far from being eternal, what will result as it is recreated in other communities of which the students are members no one can say until it happens. This reevaluation of norms in light of their consequences is another of the aspects of a democratic process that is not found in hierarchical models, which dispense 'eternal' norms 'universally' understood. This is the theoretical basis for not just listening to, but taking seriously, the contributions of each member of the group. Students and teachers alike already have moral values. They do not need to interact with the group democratically to bring their own personal values more in line with 'eternal' ones, although this is one means of seeming to do so. The Red Cells in China during Mao's reign, for instance, were quite effective in reeducating the individual's norms to the predetermined, official standards of a just society. What the democratic group situation gives them that no authoritarian system could, is the opportunity to learn how no one has a monopoly on what is a moral value, that noncoercive communities are built through cooperation, and that learning to work together means reevaluating one's values in relation to others' so that the community will work.

The unpleasant practical consequences of trying to impose one's values on the group are immediately evident. The pleasures of participating for someone who has been alienated from their school surroundings is also immediate and palpable. But it is deluding ourselves to think that the more harmonious community which emerges is a result of individuals replacing their self-centered, immature values by 'universal' ones like 'justice' and 'community'. They are learning the connections of certain means to ends, and since the experience is rewarding, it is hoped that they will try to recreate the structure in other circumstances. If, instead, they think that they are learning that their moral norms were false or immature and now they have adopted mature, eternal, universal ones, then it is likely that they will become more, not less, authoritarian in their interactions with others. Dewey explores in detail this connection of belief in absolute values with authoritarianism and of in-principle revisable moral judgments made "on the basis of public, objective and shared consequences" with the spirit of cooperation in *The Quest for Certainty* (1929, p. 47).

The democratic process may or may not lead to less absolute certainty about the universality of norms, although it is notorious that those who deal sympathetically on a day to day basis with people having diverse cultural, ethnic, religious, or political norms of morality tend to be less rigid in insisting that they alone have access to eternal norms. But the operative word is 'sympathetic'. One can learn to be more rigid and autocratic if one sees others as inferiors. By learning to treat respectfully others for whom they may not initially care, the student participants also learn to respect what others say. Thus, students' tolerance for diversity may enlarge. Another issue that emerges is also one central to feminist discourse, namely, are the members of the 'just' community learning to get along by modifying their own insights and moral stances to adopt some 'universal,' shared norms? Or are they strengthening their own uniqueness through learning to value the unique perspectives of others without seeing it as a threat to their own?

CONTEXTUALISM AND FEMINISM

Relativistic approaches to morals entail the unwanted consequence that no one could logically demand that it is a moral duty to extend to others the conditions of one's own well-being. On the other hand, universalist and necessitarian approaches to morals ignore as irrelevant the particularity of persons and historical groups and the fortuitousness present in day to day living. But these are not the only two options. In classical American philosophy values are categorized as relative to context but not relativistic, as applying to more situations than those in which they initially arose without falling into a false universalism, and as being objectively identifiable despite their origins in the uniqueness of each subject within a shared community. John Dewey developed this perspective in the greatest detail, but the pattern of his thinking can be gathered from a few quotes. In "Context and Thought" he says that "neglect of context is the greatest single disaster which philosophic thinking can incur" (Dewey 1960, p. 98). Philosophers should aim at criticizing, organizing, testing the internal coherence of, and making explicit the consequences of, the "body of beliefs and of institutions and practices allied to them" at any given time in order to develop values, understood as a projection of "a new perspective which leads to new surveys of possibilities" (Dewey 1960, pp. 106-107).

Neglect of context has prevented thinkers from realizing that "individuality in a social and moral sense" is not a given but an achievement. "It means initiative, incentiveness, varied resourcefulness, assumption of responsibility in choice of belief and conduct. . . . As achievements, they are not absolute but relative to the use that is to be made of them. And this use varies with the environment" (Dewey 1977, p. 189). Moral law is not an eternal set of principles, but "is a formula of the way to respond when specified conditions present themselves" (Dewey 1977, p. 170). Such formulas have been derived experientially, but are nonetheless objectively grounded. "Any survey of the experiences in which ends-in-view are formed, and in which earlier impulsive tendencies are shaped through deliberation into a *chosen* desire, reveals that the object finally valued as an end to be reached is determined in its concrete makeup by appraisal of existing conditions as means" (Dewey 1977, p. 176). Insofar as universalism is retained as a value, it is a goal to be achieved, not a pre-condition. "Communication, sharing, joint participation are the only actual ways of universalizing the moral law and end" (Dewey 1977, p. 195).

This perspective could be characterized as a variant of 'contextualism' or 'constructivism,' and Nona Lyons, Barbara Houston, and Nel Noddings all provide arguments supporting a feminist case for such a perspective (this volume). Lyons says that on the model that "all knowledge is contextual and constructed," then women, too, "are 'constructionists,' capable also of 'making theory.'"

For Lyons contextualism means paying more attention to women's care responses, since we already overemphasize the justice model. In this she supports Noddings' valorization of the female. Noddings (this volume) urges us to "analyze the structures and practices of our society from the perspective of women's experiences and begin the process of constructing a genuinely universal interpretation of culture." Like Houston, Noddings recognizes that the so-called equity model is actually a model developed from masculine perspectives and therefore promotes domination and oppression. But Houston (this volume) draws a very different conclusion from this insight. She warns against a premature move from an empirical claim of caring to a normative injunction. We should raise the question of what accounts for women's preference for care and what results from this orientation. By linking the valuing of caring with women's "historical context

[and] the material conditions of most women's lives," she shows how men's inculcation of this as a value for women has contributed and continues to contribute to "women's condition of subordination." Houston uses a broader notion of 'context' than Lyons's in that it includes the economic, social and political contexts in and through which women make moral decisions.

In a world in which women are exploited and dominated precisely through socializing them to unilaterally care for and service men and men's interests, it is not enough to try to educate men to also care. Women have to reconsider and re-evaluate their commitment to caring and learn to develop a strong sense of self and be motivated "to correct injustices they suffer." Women's and men's very different socialization and access to power means that the features of their moral development will and ought to differ accordingly. If it is true that society already contributes to an autonomous sense of self as a defining characteristic of the female, then this would constitute prima facie evidence that moral education should seek to develop those aspects of our ideal of humanity that the socialization process neglects with such dire consequences, that is, more autonomy for women and more connectedness for men.

GENDER-SPECIFIC OR GENDER-NEUTRAL VALUES

Noddings (this volume) quotes William James's "The Moral Equivalent of War" as instantiating the stereotype of the male warrior code, but what she does not point out is that James appeals to this model precisely to subvert it.[2] Since men's self-image in the nineteenth century—as in our own—was tied to a warrior model, James appealed to this socially constructed and reinforced model of masculinity as a gambit to redefine 'fighting' from its primary denotation of physical combat to its metaphorical sense of 'fighting' for values by peaceful means. In fact he was trying to bridge the chasm that Victorians constructed between manly 'warriors' and womanly 'moralists' by arguing that it was masculine to be a fighter for morality. That he did not extend the same reversal to women is not surprising since he was a pacifist and condemned war as a means of settling disputes. Furthermore, far from denying the heroism contained in women's experience of mothering, as Noddings claims, James frequently extolled it in glowing terms and enjoined it as model to be emulated (James 1981, pp. 1,055-1,056; James 1920, pp. 210-211). For me, this only indicates that he was unable to free himself from the Victorian stereotypes of masculinity and femininity, since—unless great care is exercised in the terms of the explanation—the glorification of motherhood as the source of women's strength reinforces a debilitating stereotype rather than being its antidote. But as a general practice James encouraged openness to perspectives neglected because of a bias in another direction. Thus, he urged philosophers and theologians to incorporate the findings of science into their outlook and scientists to take seriously feelings and values.

I agree with Noddings that James's model of an "ideal type of human character," which he says has historically been thought to be instantiated in one of three types, the saint, the knight, or the gentleman, was drawn from male experience (James 1985, p. 297). He explicitly talks about what constitutes "a certain type of man," namely, "the best man absolutely," and this heroic attitude is contrasted with "effeminacy." But then it is all the more remarkable that, despite being saddled with Victorian stereotypes and working out of his own masculine experiences, he reaches the conclusions that he does. Let us begin by recognizing his point of view and assume that he is primarily talking as a man to other men. First of all, he denies the legitimacy of appealing to "one intrinsically ideal type," even though this conception is "supposed by most persons." According to his radically empiricist philosophy "all ideals are matters of relation." Rather than an uncritical acceptance of an abstract, universal ideality he argues that we should turn to "the actual situation" and "particular circumstances" to discover the superiority of one type of conduct to another (James 1985, p. 298). He has already criticized the warrior mentality as barbarically destructive and irrational and praises only that aspect of war that encourages the "strenuous life and heroism" (James 1985, p. 292). But he is not willing to achieve these values at the cost that war exacts and therefore he searches for its "moral equivalent." Instead of "crushing weaker peoples," the heroic strenuousness he advocates is better modeled on that required in voluntarily adopting poverty, because such freedom from material attachments would enable men to stop being the "propagators of corruption" and instead "help to set free our generation" to devote themselves "to unpopular causes" (James 1985, p. 293).

He then turns to women for a better model, since their power lies not in brute force, but, like the saint, in "gentleness in beauty" (James 1985, p. 296). Although in popular imagination such moral strength seems no match for the warrior's physical strength, James argues that it can actually be more effective. A society that lived out the warrior ideal would destroy itself through unbridled aggressiveness. The saint as hero better realizes both the means to and the end of a perfect society, which is conceived as one "in which there would be no aggressiveness, but only sympathy and fairness" (James 1985, p. 298). Furthermore we already have living examples on a small scale of what we are aiming for on a large scale: "any small community of true friends now realizes such a society." His reconstruction of men's ideal of a properly masculine heroic strength thus involves a double strategy: first of all, showing that brute force is less effective than peaceful means of combatting evil of all kinds, and secondly, that a moral reconstruction of society can be at least as exciting as the martial arts. This double strategy of both developing a moral ideal that will fire a man's imagination and provide motive power and demonstrating its usefulness as a practical recourse and not merely an unrealistic ideal is based on his analysis of practical rationality as constituted by interactive aesthetic and practical aspects.

In turning from an abstract ideal of community to our actual societies we find that the exact mix of characteristics which will both be practically livable and still heroically ideal can vary a great deal, just as the situations vary. What is called for in one situation is not neccessarily transferable to a different one, even though we can agree in a preliminary way what the characteristics are that are most admirable. In uncovering the destructiveness of central concepts of masculinity that his society uncritically accepted and reconstructing a model of masculinity that incorporated what was commonly assigned to femininity, James provides us with a model of analysis that is arguably worth appropriating, once it is purged of those "special historic manifestations" that in hindsight are no longer acceptable to us (James 1985, p. 295). Finally, it is significant that in holding up heroic, saintly models for emulation he includes both men and women, especially if one is assuming, as Noddings does, that he is speaking as a man. By substituting the living model of a "community of true friends" that is small enough to be interactive for the oppressive machismo of the male warrior model, he is already proposing nonsexist explanations that can be profitably developed further by those of us for whom this move is central, not peripheral.

SYMPATHETIC CARING AS AN ORIGIN OF VALUES

In closing I would like to propose an ethical perspective that places something very like care at the center of its value system as a model that other feminists might also find worthwhile reconstructing in the light of our present-day knowledge and interests. It is found in William James's (1983) "On a Certain Blindness in Human Beings," where he argues that judgments of worth have their origins in feeling. If we had no feelings ideals would not have any significance for us and we would not discriminate them into values worth pursuing. But although feeling is a necessary condition, it is not a sufficient one, because we must still determine which of our predilections ought to be pursued in preference to others.

Since we are practical beings our own situations and duties are of intense and constant interest, but we do not generally expect others to attach such importance to what concerns our inner life. Like us, they have their own vital interests. We therefore often misjudge the significance of lives different from our own. "Hence the falsity of our judgments, so far as they presume to decide in an absolute way on the values of other person's conditions or ideals" (James 1983, p. 132). This congenital blindness toward the feelings of peoples and creatures different from ourselves is the greatest obstacle to the ethical life. Without this basic sympathy we would have no motive for attributing an ideality to a way of life alien to our own. Since we are finite and practical creatures, the pursuit of those duties which constitute our vocation or situation in life tends toward dulling our sensitivity to the vital centers which animate others. It takes both a leap of the imagination and determined effort to recognize and sympathize with "the higher vision of inner significance" of others, and to find "a new centre and a new perspective" extending the original boundaries of our own felt interests (James 1983, p. 138).

This sympathy goes beyond tolerance because it seeks to gain insight into the individuated worlds of experience of others and the values they hold that make these worlds cohere. This insight is only available from a perspective of caring. James calls it a "sympathetic, concrete observation" that understands more than is visible to disinterested scrutiny. It is a necessary precondition for concrete judgments of justice, as he argues in "The Moral Philosopher and the Moral Life" (James 1979). Without it justice is either so abstract that its practical meaning must still be determined through a process such as "sympathetic concrete observation," that is, observation, reflection, appraisal, instantiation, and revision, or it merely imposes, with little regard to the specificity of the situation, a rigid moral outlook which is claimed to be universal, but actually incorporates a particular world view and code of values.

No philosophy of ethics is possible on the traditional model seeking to ground a system of abstract rules deduced from unrevisable, universal moral imperatives, "for every real dilemma is in literal strictness a unique situation; and the exact combination of ideals realized and ideals disappointed which each decision creates is always a universe without a precedent, and for which no adequate previous rule exists" (James 1979, p. 158). This does not deny that in every actual moral deliberation predetermined rules and judgments of value have a vital role to play. But unless these rules and valuations themselves undergo intelligent modification through operational thinking, the gap between transcendent values and everyday life will eventually be so great as to negate any directive function. According to Dewey (1929 p. 273) "what is needed is intelligent examination of the consequences that are actually affected by inherited institutions and customs, in order that there may be intelligent consideration of the ways in which they are to be intentionally modified in behalf of generation of different consequences."

This insistence on the irreducible value of each person's experience is also central to feminist theory. Both outlooks recognize that in this imperfect world of ours there are no guarantees that the moral choices we make are the right ones, and insists that a place be found for each one's values in the total universe of values, insofar as this is possible. Since women, along with other oppressed groups, have suffered from the imposition of values falsely labeled universal, but developed in ignorance of our experiences, the criterion James gives for identifying mistaken moral choices should awaken curiosity about the possibility of appropriating his ethical outlook. He says that when we err "the cries of the wounded will inform [us] of the fact" (James 1979, p. 158).

NOTES

1. See John Dewey (1983) on the generic traits of existence. A good overview of this theme, including what is found in his other works, is provided by Hawn and Boydston (1970 pp. 43-48). See also his definition of "situation" or "context" (Dewey 1963, pp. 43-44).

2. Noddings refers to the passage mentioning "the moral equivalent of war" in *The varieties of religious experience* (James 1985). The longer essay with this title can be found in *Essays in religion and morality* (James 1982). For the connection between the two, see James (1982, pp. 195, n. 1621 and pp. 251ff.). My remarks refer to both.

REFERENCES

Beauvoir, S. de. (1974). *The second sex*. New York: Vintage Books.

Bebeau, M. J., and Brabeck, M. M. (1987). Integrating care and justice issues in professional moral education: A gender perspective. *Journal of Moral Education* 16:189-203.

Dewey, J. (1929). *The quest for certainty* (Chap. 10). New York: Minton, Balch.

_____ . (1946). *The problems of men*. New York: Philosophical Library.

_____ . (1957). *Human nature and conduct*. New York: Modern Library.

_____ . (1960). Context and thought. In *On experience, nature, and freedom*, pp. 88-110, ed. Richard J. Bernstein. Indianapolis: The Liberal Arts Press.

_____ . (1963). *Experience and education*. New York: Collier Books.

_____ . (1977). The construction of good (pp. 153-175); Propositions of Appraisal (pp. 176-184); Reconstruction as affecting social philosophy (pp. 185-196). In *John Dewey: The essential writings*, ed. David Sidorsky. New York: Harper Torchbooks.

_____ . (1983). *The later works of John Dewey. Vol. I: 1925. Experience and nature*. Carbondale, Illinois: Southern Illinois University Press.

Gilligan, C. (1982). *In a different voice: Psychological theory and women's development*. Cambridge, Mass.: Harvard University Press.

Hawn, L. E., and Boydston, J. A., eds. (1970). *Guide to the works of John Dewey*. Carbondale, Ill.: Southern Illinois University Press.

James, W. (1920). *The letters of William James, Vol. 1*. Ed. Henry James. Boston: The Atlantic Monthly Press.

_____ . (1979). The moral philosopher and the moral life. *The will to believe* (pp. 141-162). Cambridge, Mass.: Harvard University Press.

———— . (1981). *The principles of psychology*, vol. 2. Cambridge: Harvard University Press.

———— . (1982). The moral equivalent of war. In *Essays in religion and morality* (pp. 162-173). Cambridge, Mass.: Harvard University Press.

———— . (1983). On a certain blindness in human beings. In *Talks to teachers on psychology* (pp. 132-149). Cambridge, Mass.: Harvard University Press.

———— . (1985). *The varieties of religious experience*. Cambridge, Mass.: Harvard University Press.

Seigfried, C. Haddock. (1982). Vagueness and the adequacy of concepts. *Philosophy Today* (Winter):357-367.

———— . (1984). Gender-specific values. *The Philosophical Forum* 15: 425-442.

———— . (1985). Second sex: Second thoughts. *Women's Studies International Forum* 8:219-229.

5

Prolegomena to Future Caring

Barbara Houston

> Until we can understand the assumptions in which we are drenched, we
> cannot know ourselves.
>
> Adrienne Rich (1979)

INTRODUCTION

When John Stuart Mill was asked the question, "What is the nature of
Woman?" he replied to this effect: "I can hardly say, women themselves
will have to tell us." Happily, at this point in history, there are some women
who are telling us what woman's moral nature is. In this chapter I will
examine the work of two of these women, Carol Gilligan (1982) and Nel
Noddings (1984). (All references to these two authors are from these
works.) Both have undertaken to describe women's moral thinking and the
implications of their insights for ethics, for theories of moral development,
and for theories of moral education.

As a woman I feel myself enormously indebted to both Carol Gilligan and
Nel Noddings for they have each, in different ways, helped to articulate
dimensions of my moral thinking and feeling which have not been formalized
in standard ethical theories. In attending closely to the substance of women's
experiences they have seen and made visible to me realms of moral activity
which have gone unnoticed or have been devalued and dismissed in ethical
theories which purport to be about all human moral experience.

The standard ethical theories which have been influential in shaping my own
philosophical outlook are those that have given me some leaning toward
Platonic assumptions about ideals, a Kantian commitment to the value of
persons as ends in themselves, a Rawlsian sense of justice as fairness, and, thus,
some initial sympathy with Kohlberg's view of moral development.

However, within these theories, there have been, as Annette Baier puts it,
"only hand waves concerning our proper attitude to our children, to the ill,

This chapter has benefited from my discussions with Barbara Brockelman, Nel
Noddings, and especially Ann Diller. I am grateful to them for their support and
encouragement.

to our relatives, friends and lovers" (Baier 1985, p. 55). These "special relations," as they are called, are often passed over in ethical theories which take justice, fairness or impartiality as the central moral value. Consider Kurt Baier's remark about the "moral point of view" and when it is appropriately adopted:

I take it that moral reasoning comes into the picture only when the goals of individuals come into conflict with one another. For only then is there a need for reasons . . . designed to adjudicate between conflicting needs, wants and aspirations of different individuals. I assume then that the existence of moral reasoning presuppose(s) the normal interactions between persons (Baier 1965, p. 110).

These so-called "special relations" and "normal interactions between persons" have constituted the major part of women's work. Within a woman's perspective, the relatedness that lies at the heart of our "normal interactions with persons" is not something that just occurs, it already represents some sort of moral achievement. This relatedness requires a sustained moral activity and moral attention which is called caring.

Traditionally women have been charged with the responsibility for nurturing and caring for others, especially the young, the old, the ill, and those in intimate relation with them. Unhappily this labor, like housework, seems invisible if done well. But now Gilligan, a psychologist, and Noddings, a philosopher, have undertaken an exploration of the moral activity of caring. They begin to make this moral labor visible and if they are correct, a very different sort of ethics may be generated by this moral labor. Joining them in their exploration of an ethics of care, I raise certain questions and unresolved puzzles that arise as I reflect on the care perspective and think about possible formulations for a coherent system of ethics based on it.

I am interested in the problems associated with a coherent formulation of an ethics of care, not the empirical question of whether there are sex differences in the use of this morality. While both Noddings and Gilligan believe care to be a morality that is predominant among women, both express doubts about the empirical thesis that it belongs only to women. Certainly neither of them believes that this morality cannot belong to men, and for the purposes of assessing it as a morality, this is the critical assumption.

Kurt Baier (1965) reminds us that whatever else a morality is, it has to be accessible for everyone. He accurately points out the one sense in which morality is clearly characterized by universality.

Morality is not the preserve of an oppressed or privileged class or individual. . . . An esoteric code, a set of precepts known only to the initiated and perhaps jealously concealed from outsiders, can at best be a religion, not a morality. . . . "Thou shalt not kill, but it is a secret" is absurd. 'Esoteric morality' is a contradiction in terms (Baier 1965, p. 101).

Drawing out the implications of this feature of universality, Baier rightly reminds us that a morality must be teachable; not just learnable, but teachable.[1] Noddings and Gilligan both allow that an ethics of care could be taught to men, and hence this minimal conceptual requirement of the ethics of care being a morality are satisfied.

One further note. In posing my puzzles and queries I shall adopt the point of view of women. I agree with Gilligan and Noddings that this has too seldom been the perspective taken in assessing or developing ethical theories. Did Aristotle ask Mrs. Aristotle what she thought of his ethics?[2] It's highly unlikely, since he thought the chief virtues of a woman were silence and obedience. Undoubtedly his ethics would be quite different if he had asked Mrs. Aristotle what she thought about it. Given that the perspective of women has rarely, if ever, been the perspective employed in testing ethical theories, in the present historical circumstances it can hardly be a biased way to proceed.

AN ETHICS OF CARE: ITS SUBJECT MATTER, ITS FORMULATION

We do not yet have a definitive formulation of an ethics of care, but Gilligan and Noddings agree on features of the ethics. First, as I have mentioned, one of the chief virtues of an ethics of care is that it includes within the moral realm activities which standard theories exclude or devalue. It is an ethics which claims that the point of morality is to establish a world in which we remain in relation with one another. Within Gilligan's "care orientation" and within Noddings' more formal theory, caring is taken to be the very foundation of the ethical.

Eschewing the focus of other recent moral theorists on judgment making, Noddings asks us to reorient our attention to what she calls the moral attitude. For her the basic question of ethics is, "How am I to meet the other morally?" (p. 201). Her answer is, "One must meet the other as one-caring. From this requirement there is no escape for one who would be moral" (p. 201).

To understand both Gilligan's and Noddings' work, one must recognize that relatedness is a fact of human existence which an ethics of care endows with moral significance. Other ethical theories endow different facts of our experience with moral significance: for example, our alleged egoism, our conflict of interests with others, or our capacity to experience pleasure and pain. Gilligan and Noddings both recognize that caring is most fundamentally a *relation*. Noddings is particularly emphatic in claiming that caring is not a unilateral action; caring is something that is completed in the cared-for. As Noddings puts it, the attitude of the one-caring must be received and completed in the cared-for. She notes that, "The receiving of the caring may be accomplished in a disclosure of [the cared-for's] own subjective experience in direct response to the one-caring or by a happy and vigorous pursuit of his own projects" (p. 151).

Noddings describes caring primarily from the point of view of the one-caring. From this perspective caring is seen to have two distinctive features: engrossment and motivational displacement. Engrossment is characterized as a receptive mode of consciousness in which "we receive what is there as nearly as possible without evaluation or assessment" (p. 34). Clarifying what she means by motivational displacement, Noddings claims that we apprehend the other's reality so that, "when we see the other's reality as a possibility for me, we must act to eliminate the intolerable, to reduce the pain, to fill the need to actualize the dream" (p. 14). Thus, caring involves more than feeling *with* someone; it also involves a motivational shift. "My motive energy flows towards the other and perhaps, . . . towards his ends" (p. 33).

The caring attitude may be summed up as a "readiness to bestow and spend oneself and make oneself available" (p. 19). In caring, Noddings says, there is "a total conveyance of the self to the other" (p. 61). For both Gilligan and Noddings caring is also a commitment to an attitude that keeps one responsive to others.

From within the ethics of care we have generated the important imperatives, "always meet the other as one-caring," and "maintain and enhance the caring relation." As we listen to the women in Gilligan's studies, these imperatives are heeded. These women do take seriously their obligation to meet the other as one-caring and to maintain and enhance those relations in which they act as ones-caring. As Gilligan notes, they undertake to resolve conflicts by maintaining or strengthening their connections with those with whom they are in conflict; when presented with dilemmas of conflict, they vigorously search for solutions which are of this nature. This approach to solving moral problems has been called by Gilligan "the method of inclusion." In a very general sense, we may say that "the care orientation" simply invites us to identify the needs of persons "in conflict" and create solutions to meet them.

CAN AN ETHICS OF CARE AVOID SELF-SACRIFICE?

When I reflect on the history of women, I realize how much our caring has nurtured and empowered others. I see how good it has been, for others. However, I also see how terribly costly it has been for women. And so the first question that arises for me is one that arises for many of Gilligan's subjects. Can an ethics of care avoid self-sacrifice?

There are different ways to put this question that arises from my own "living doubt" about the ethics of care as described by Gilligan and Noddings. Claudia Card (1985), for example, asks it this way: "Is Gilligan picking up on something Nietzsche identified as a 'slave morality'?" (p. 6)[3] One might also ask the question in such a way as to reveal more obviously its political nature: Has women's 'ethics of care' contributed to women's powerlessness vis-à-vis men over the centuries? Is it a morality that contributes to or augments women's oppression?

Within Gilligan's care orientation, there is an obvious struggle with this question, in its individualistic form if not in its political form. For some of her research subjects a clear recognition emerges that they have responsibilities to care for themselves. At the final "stage" in Gilligan's care orientation women realize that "responsiveness to self and responsiveness to others are connected rather than opposed" (p. 61). In Noddings's work I also find a clear awareness of the risks and dangers to the self in caring for others and hence some recognition that it is necessary to care for the self if one is to maintain oneself as one-caring. However, in neither work do I find what I take to be a clear answer to the question concerning self-sacrifice. Instead, at the heart of the justification process, describing just how responsiveness to self and responsiveness to others are related, I find a highly unsettling ambiguity concerning the moral worth of persons.

The first and most striking feature of the justification process is that the presumption is in favor of caring and it is *not-caring* that requires justification. This is a dramatic reversal of the tenet in most ethical theories which accepts the presumption of self-interest and requires a justification of altruism.

There appear to be only two acceptable reasons for not caring: (1) it will interfere with my realizing my obligations to those for whom I already care; and (2) it will cause harm to my physical or ethical self, that is, to my self as one-caring (Noddings, 1984, p. 100). Thus, we see reflected at the heart of an ethics of care the observation made by Gilligan that the individual defines herself and judges herself in terms of her ability to care. Since an ethics of care takes as its ontology persons-in-relation and endows this fact of human relatedness with moral significance, the attribution of moral worth to persons appears to apply to them only as one-caring. The unconditional worth of the *cared for* is unequivocally assumed by Gilligan's subjects and by Noddings. They assume that the needs of others make claims upon our care which can only be ignored if we have justification. It is less obvious that unconditional value is assumed for the one-caring. As long as this ambiguity remains, we cannot be assured that the ethics of care will assist women in avoiding self-sacrifice. Nor can we be sure that the ethics of care will avoid the subordination of the interests of women, as a group, to the interests of other groups, for example, men and children.

If the one-caring sees her moral worth as wholly dependent upon her capacity to care for others, or as contingent upon being in relation then she may remain as one-caring in relations that are harmful to her. Thus, I suggest a formalized ethics of care must answer a question of clarification: Within an ethics of care does the moral worth of a woman arise solely from her being in a caring relation? To put it another way, Do my obligations to care for myself, as a woman, arise wholly out of my caring relations with others? When put in their political form, with the interests of women as a group in mind, the questions of clarifications might be these: Does the value of women rest in their capacity to care for others? Do women's moral obligations to attend to the interests of women as a group arise wholly out of women's service role vis-à-vis other groups in society?

The ambiguity concerning these matters in the ethics of care as it is articulated by Gilligan and Noddings is a serious matter inasmuch as it is women's morality we are discussing. Traditionally women's role has been that of service to others and women's value has been seen to rest here. Indeed, it is precisely because there is strong precedence for defining woman as a "helpmate to man" that we need to query whether the allegedly distinctive morality of women challenges this notion.

Again, it is important to notice that it is the historical context, the material conditions of most women's lives, that prompts us to press for clear, unequivocal answers to these questions. Most women's lives are governed by a sexual division of labor that overrides other differences among them. As Marilyn Frye (1983) notes, women of all races and classes are together in "a ghetto of sorts." There is, as she notes, a woman's place that is defined by function and the function is "the service of men and men's interests as men define them, which includes the bearing and rearing of children" (Frye 1983, p. 9). Granted, the details and working conditions of women's lives vary by race and class because men of different races and classes have different interests and perceive their interests and needs differently. However, there are, as Frye observes, some predictable constants:

Whether in lower, middle or upper class homes or work situations, women's service work always includes personal service (the work of maids, butlers, cooks, personal secretaries), sexual service (including provision for his genital sexual needs and bearing his children, but also including "being nice," "being attractive for him," etc.) and ego service (encouragement, support, praise, attention) (Frye 1983, p. 9).

Thus, there is a good reason to wonder whether an ethics of care deriving from women's moral practices in the context of oppressive conditions will reflect the notions of the worth of women consistent with women's condition of subordination.

THE RELATION BETWEEN WORTHY CARING RELATIONS AND THE SOCIAL CONTEXT

The second issue I want to raise concerns the danger of valuing caring relations separate from the economic, political, and social context in which they occur. I worry that too little attention is paid within the ethics of care to the fact that social contexts can systematically deform caring relations and render caring ineffective.

I want to develop this point by considering an actual example of a lesson in the ethics of care which I think is quite common to the moral education of most young girls. Ellen Goodman in one of her columns gives us a good description of the lesson and her own ambivalence about it.

The little girl doesn't understand. A boy in her first grade class has selected her as his recess quarry. All week he has pursued her, capturing her scarf, circling her with it, threatening to tie her up.

The look on her face as she tells us this is puzzled and upset. My friend who is her mother . . . explains to the girl, "that's because he likes you." But she still doesn't understand.

Then the mother turns to Ellen Goodman in frustration and says, "Tell her." Ellen Goodman writes:

I begin to form the analysis in my mind. I will tell her how the boy wants attention, doesn't know how to ask for it, only knows how to grab for it, confuses aggression with affection. . . (Goodman 1982).

But then Ellen Goodman stops for she hears inside her head "an echo of a hundred generations of women interpreting males to their daughters." We might say "an echo of a hundred generations of women" teaching their daughters the ethics of care. And she finds herself, as I do, with some reluctance to pass on this legacy, wary of teaching the little girl the ethics of care. Perhaps we all feel some ambivalence about the lesson, yet it is instructive to explore the ambivalence and to examine why we can take this to be a reasonable lesson to give a young girl in the ethics of care.

Noddings, brilliantly, notices that one of the crucial responsibilities the one-caring takes on is the nurturance of the goodness of the cared-for. In committing ourselves to the task of furthering another's well-being, we recognize that nurturance of the ethical self of the cared-for is an important, if not *the* important, dimension of our caretaking. This dimension of care generates certain prescriptions for us. Three of the ones Noddings describes might be called:

1. The Prescription of Good Motive Attribution: "the one-caring should attribute the best possible motive consonant with reality to the cared-for" (p. 103).[4]
2. The Prescription to Preserve Future Caring: If the one-caring should find that she fails to care any more, "she must not do anything which would jeopardize the caring others might have for him" (p. 115).
3. The Prescription of Behaving-As-If: When the one-caring is, in turn, the one cared-for and yet fails to experience the caring attitude from the one presumed caring for her, she should nevertheless act as if she received caring. The cared-for

acts in this way in order to maintain the relation and to induce the one-caring to genuinely feel the caring attitude (p. 76).[5]

We can see, I think, how the lesson I described entails teaching the little girl these prescriptions. Most obviously the lesson *directly* teaches her to presume a good motive, but we can also see how she would indirectly learn the other two prescriptions if we consider how she might behave toward this boy in the future. We can imagine that she might not report him to school officials who would discipline him, or she might think she should not tell his parents or even her own parents who might think badly of him. The next time he does it, she may not protest to him as much as she wants to. She may not let him know how much it hurts her, or how angry it makes her when he behaves as he does.

Now, among some caring relations, such as those mothers have with their children, these tenets of an ethics of care are understandable and desirable. Indeed they appear to describe precisely the kind of moral thinking that goes into good caring for children. All the tenets urge us to see the cared-for in the best possible light, and we can grant that this is essential in helping children (and others) to realize their best self. Further, the asymmetry of power relations within the context of women caring for children are such that following these tenets need not render women vulnerable in any undesirable way. However, the employment of these tenets without any prescription for mutuality in other kinds of caring relationships means that the ethics recommends moral strategies which call for self-sacrifice on the part of girls and women within present economic, social, and political contexts. Let me explain.

In considering these prescriptions, I was struck by how they seemed to explain in part what reduces the ability of girls and women to resist or to avoid physical and sexual abuse. These prescriptions may also interfere with our willingness to seek help when we have been abused. The literature on this social problem reveals that women are the ones who feel guilty about their abuse; women are the ones who feel they have not managed the relationship well; we do not speak out for fear of not being believed, for fear of being thought bad, for fear of causing trouble for the men involved. Unhappily, our fears are realistic. The abusive men (ranging from fathers, other men in the family, to professors and doctors placed in the public role of caretakers) are protected. Does this misplaced protection have its root in a one-sided ethics of care?

I think it does, partly, for the ethics gives us prescriptions which are so easily rendered problematic *if there is within the ethics* no clear, unambiguous, independent moral worth assigned to the one caring, or some clear directives concerning the importance of the interests of women. Consider how these presumptions might interconnect to immobilize the one caring in relations that are destructive to her.

If my caring relation is one that has built into it some expectation that it is to persist, then the ethics encourages me to act as though I am cared for when I am not. This behaving-as-if, practiced often enough, can deceive me as well as the one presumed caring. The matter is enormously complicated by the fact that I am also to attribute to the cared-for, "the best possible motive consonant with reality." This can help rationalize any behavior toward me that is perceived as destructive, in a way that can make me *at least unsure* that others have acted badly toward me. Finally, publicly acknowledging that others have not been caring for me, indeed have been abusive toward me, is certainly a way of closing off the possibility of future caring for them that is something else the ethics forbids except in the most extreme cases.

We can now imagine, and some of us may know firsthand, how these tenets of an ethics of care can induce a moral paralysis in the one-caring in situations in which she needs to act to protect herself. Although the ethic says that we may abandon our caring attitude when our physical or ethical self is in danger, the fact is that our society so structures the power relations between the genders that *for women*, the protection of our physical self is put in conflict with the protection of our ethical self. It is because our society puts the protection of these selves in conflict that women's caring often becomes distorted, defective, harmful to us, and frequently even to the cared-for (Blum et al., 1979).

The little girl lives in a society in which men are often violent toward women. She lives in a society in which girls and women are devalued. She lives in a society in which girls and women are expected to be caring toward boys and men even when it is to their own detriment; they are expected to be trusting even when they have strong reasons to distrust. This knowledge of the political and social context makes me reluctant about the lesson. The social structures of the society make it positively *dangerous* to teach this little girl to presume the best motive consonant with reality in this case. It may be something that the boy's parents should utilize in teaching him. But this little girl needs to be encouraged to express her own anger at what has occurred. She needs to be taught that even if the boy acted this way out of some liking for her, it is still unacceptable.

But matters are even more complex, for the little girl has also to be made aware that others may chastise her for making "much ado about nothing," for not recognizing that "boys will be boys," and that part of her *role* is to accept it with good humor. For later, as Ellen Goodman points out, as an adult woman she will be expected to explain men's behavior to others, to interpret for him in social relationships and this too is part of what we are supposed to teach her when we teach her why the boy did what he did. We are to initiate her into a "cult of communication," to help her acquire the knowledge and grace she needs to fulfill her role as an adult woman, as a mother.

Ellen Goodman (1982) looks at her friend, the little girl's mother and sees

a woman . . . admirably skilled in the task of transmitting one person's ideas and feelings to another. Indeed, she operates the switchboard of her family home.

The people in her home communicate through her. She delivers peace messages from one child to another. Softens ultimatums from father to son; explains the daughter to the father. Under her constant monitoring, the communication lines are kept open; one person stays plugged to the next.

But she again asks herself a question which explains more of her reluctance to give the girl the lesson:

[S]ometimes I wonder whether she has kept all these people together or kept them apart. Does she make it easier for them to understand each other, or does she actually stand between them, holding all the wires in her hands?

Thus, we can see that in this small lesson in the ethics of care lies a great deal of female socialization into women's roles in society. This too needs to be overtly challenged or the little girl will know only that she hasn't handled it "right" because of the way others view her when she feels entitled to be angry.

Now it might be argued that in some sense an ethics of care as formulated by Gilligan and Noddings can easily handle this problem inasmuch as their ethics of care urges us to pay close attention to the context in which we make our moral decisions. They are the first to claim that any presumptions or rules or tenets are merely suggestive guidelines. However, I am not wholly reassured by this. The directive to attend to the context does not tell us what we are to count as the context, nor does it tell us what in the context we should attend to.

The point I am making here is a very general one which has been made often by feminist commentators. For example, Jean Grimshaw describes a "politics of caring" (1986, p. 216). Historically, and within our present society, appeals to caring are sometimes used oppressively and in a manner that disguises social relationships of exploitation and domination, especially, but not only, between women and men. Often accusations of failure to care are directed at women in a way which serves to divert attention from the issues of women's subordination to men, or from certain injustices women suffer. For example, women who seek some time, privacy, or increased control over their lives are often accused by their husband or families of not caring; women are accused of man-hating if they propose women's studies programs or the need for women-only space; women who lobby for equal pay for work of equal value are bizarrely accused of lesbianism or denying men sexual access to them (Atkinson 1974).

Gilligan's answer to the dilemma posed by a conflict of interest between the one-caring and the one-cared for is to insist that, in its most mature

form, the ethics of care asserts that responsiveness to self and responsiveness to others are connected rather than opposed (Gilligan 1982, pp. 74,
149). This may suggest a useful strategy when trying to lobby for one's own
interests with those who would deny them, but I am not persuaded that it is
a helpful answer to our problem. We live in a society which charges women
with the responsibility for caring for others, especially children. Our society
is also structured so that women's interests are put in conflict with men's,
and some women's and children's interests (white, middle class) are put in
conflict with the interests of other women and children (black, lower class).
If we are to alter women's condition of exploitation, if we are to eliminate
injustices they suffer, then as Grimshaw points out, someone is going to be
deprived of something to which they are accustomed: attention, service or
amenities (Grimshaw 1986, p. 218). It will involve hardships and difficulties
for some people; for example, men may have less money, or not as great an
opportunity for better paying jobs, or less leisure time. This will be experienced by them as a lack of care. Indeed, one of the things that has to be
redistributed is women's care and some will have less caring from women.
We might want no opposition between the interests of women, as a group,
and men, as a group, and in the ideal society we might be able to arrange
things that way. But for now, interests, or at least perceived interests, are in
conflict and any attempt to alter the present conditions is going to bring
charges of a failure to care. If Gilligan's answer is to be satisfactory, it will
have to include some fuller account of conflicting interests.

I am not much more reassured by Noddings's answer to the dilemmas
posed by the "politics of caring." Her answer to this concern, as I understand it, is threefold: (1) Recognize that within the ethics of care there is a
limitation placed on caring; it is to be abandoned if it places one's physical
or ethical self in danger. (2) Recognize that there are, of course,
pathological uses of the ethics of care, but remember that the ethics cannot
be faulted for all the mistakes people make when using it. After all, as J. S.
Mill said, combine any theory with human idiocy and you will get bad
results. (3) Recognize that morality is, after all, an ideal, and that one
should expect that it may involve some degree of sacrifice.[6]

The first part of Noddings's answer appears to me to beg the question for
two reasons. First, as I have mentioned, in our current situation the protection of women's physical self is often put in conflict with the protection of
their ethical self, at least their ethical self as society defines it. Consider the
woman who goes to court to get a restraining order placed on her husband
because he is physically abusive toward her or who seeks the protection of
the police to allow her to remove some of her possessions from her home
because she is worried that her husband might kill her. Such a woman may
be told by court officials that she is a nuisance to society and (or because)
she has failed at her domestic responsibilities.

We can take Noddings to mean that we should appeal to the ethical
self—not as society defines it, not in terms of society's notion of how a

woman should care—but as Noddings defines it. If we do this, I am still not reassured that we have a safe criterion that will rescue women from their exploitative situations of caring. Noddings roots her ethical ideal of the self as one-caring in the history of caring each of us has had. In moments of uncertainty we are to appeal for guidance to our remembrances of experiences in which we were cared for. However, given women's history of oppression, given the misogyny and sexism that has pervaded our culture for centuries, given even the most conservative facts about the amount of physical and sexual abuse women have suffered and continue to suffer,[7] I am not at all confident that we can count on this bank of remembrances of caring for the people who may most often have occasion to use it. Women have not consistently been cherished and cared for, so the ideal we are to appeal to as a corrective may not work. Even if women do remember the caring, we are also bound to remember the context in which it occurred. This context attached a terrible cost to caring, a cost most often borne by our mothers and foremothers. The caring our mothers gave us may have cost them beatings, abuse, incredible hardship, the opportunities to be economically independent; it may even have cost them death. How, from this history, from this bank of remembrances of caring, are women to judge when their ethical self is legitimately in danger?

Considering Noddings's second answer to our worry, I will grant that any ethics is subject to pathological use. However, the doubts I and others have about the ethics of care cannot be simply or easily identified as a problem with those who use it rather than a problem with the ethics. Given women's history of oppression, given the unjust distribution of responsibility for caring, we might reasonably expect, among women, that the pathological use of the ethics of care will be as common as the nonpathological uses of it. Oppression, as we are reminded, is not only external, but also internal. We should expect that women are a damaged people and susceptible to a use of the ethics of care which will entrench their subordination, or at the least, not challenge it.[8]

These considerations have two consequences for our assessment of the ethics of care. First, if the ethics is a description of women's caring practices in conditions of subordination and exploitation, then it may not have clear criteria for distinguishing between legitimate and illegitimate forms of caring. Second, these considerations should alert us to implicit assumptions about the nature of the moral agents which are built into any ethics.

Annette Baier complains that traditional ethical theories have presupposed on the part of moral agents both "an equality of power and a separateness from others which is salient to women's experience of life and morality" (1986, p. 247). She pointedly remarks that since women's moral dealings are more frequently with the less powerful and the more powerful, "a code of ethics which is designed for those equal in power will be at best nonfunctional and at worst an offensive pretense of equality as a substitute for its actuality" (Baier 1986, p. 247).

The ethic of care certainly does recognize the ways in which we are inter-connected; it takes seriously moral relations with those with whom we are intimate and those who either cannot or should not achieve equality of power with us: animals, the ill, the dying, and children while still young. It recognizes our dependence upon one another for everything, including moral goodness. But it fails to address "the shifting and varying power asymmetry" among moral agents, as well as the "shifting and varying intimacy" (Baier 1986, p. 250). It fails in the way other ethical theories have failed us; it does not give us much help with "the proper attitude of the powerless to be powerful" (p. 291). Yet, as Annette Baier remarks, it is these relationships as well as those of equality which also "determine the state of moral health or corruption in which we are content to live" (1986, p. 251).

The successful use of the ethics of care as Noddings describes it presup-poses a certain kind of moral agent: one who is clear about the boundaries of the self so that she can practice the demanding task of engrossment without the loss of self being a problem for her. It presupposes an agent who has a realistic sense of her own competencies and a sense of that which she can reasonably take responsibility for so that she can separate from situations in which caring is not effective and, again, do so without a loss of self. In short, Noddings seems to presuppose the sort of self we might want for women, but which we must recognize is not a women's self for which there is much support in the culture.

Finally, I agree with Noddings that, in a sense, the point of ethics is to recognize that one's own interests are not always overriding and that, on certain occasions, they are less important than the needs of others. We need to recognize, with Gilligan and Noddings, that women's caring has been in-visible and devalued. However, we must also recognize that women's caring has been systematically appealed to in order to distract women from efforts to correct injustices they suffer ("Who will look after the children?"). Any adequate account of women's morality is going to have to show some recognition of this, and show how the ethics we propose that women adopt challenges this division of moral labor, and will not, in the present cir-cumstances, contribute to women's continued subordination.

To return to the dilemma with which we began, I recognize that there is no easy answer to the dilemma posed by the lesson in caring we are expected to give to the little girl. I feel *ambivalent* about the lesson because I can see that these presumptions or tenets of the ethics of care should not be aban-doned easily, for they reflect dimensions of trust. And trust is needed for persons to be in relation. But while it is obvious that these tenets cannot just be abandoned, it is clear that we need something more. We need within the ethics of care some clear directives about when these tenets are not ap-plicable. At the moment they presume a trust in the other that, in many cir-cumstances in which girls and women find themselves, is inappropriate or misplaced. In order to avoid these dangers, our ethics of care needs some stronger, fuller concepts of what Annette Baier (1985) calls "appropriate trust" and "proper distrust."

SOME IMPLICATIONS FOR MORAL EDUCATION

Does the differential moral experience of girls and boys, women and men carry any implications for moral development or moral education? Noddings makes the observation that, "Too often it is women who are cast in the role of one-caring and men who are cared-for" (p. 127). In considering this, she suggests that women must learn how to better maintain themselves as ones-caring, perhaps by strengthening their self-image, and men must learn to care.

One problem I see with both Noddings's and Kohlberg's approaches to moral education is that they both put women's struggle for a strong sense of self outside the moral domain. Noddings sees it as a matter of acquiring a stronger self-image and suggests that working in the public sector may help women acquire it. I think this is unlikely because to a large extent the jobs available to women in the public sector simply duplicate the roles we are expected to play in the private realm. The jobs available to us are primarily service jobs which are low paying and have low status. In these jobs we have our sense of worth only as one-caring reinforced, and our caring activity devalued.

Kohlberg and some others think that the issues often described within the care orientation are issues concerning "ego development," a matter of girls learning to "disentangle the self from conformity expectations," a matter of simply learning the ability to say "no" (Nunner-Winkler 1984, p. 357). But in failing to attend to the substance of this struggle in the case of girls and women, they fail to notice and accord it the proper moral significance.

The struggle women wage to disentangle themselves from conformity expectations is a complex one. It is in fact a fourfold struggle that is occurring. It involves:

1. A struggle to determine the worthiness both of society's expectations that we as women care for others, and of society's views about how we as women should care for others;

2. A struggle to solve an as yet unresolved moral problem concerning conflicting responsibilities to oneself (as a woman) and to others, a conflict concerning the boundary between what is morally required and what is supererogatory;

3. A struggle to articulate responsibilities, values, and ways of thinking that have not been articulated in influential ethical theories and are not publicly confirmed; and it is finally, and most poignantly;

4. A struggle to know our own moral worth in a society that systematically denies it.

In Kohlberg's scheme of development one is to move from the self-love of the egoist, in essence from the first waking of self, of one's own desires, needs, interests, wants, and an awareness of their relevance to morality, to a fully recognized moral worth accorded all persons within an ethics of justice. This may be possible for white males in this culture; a culture in which "human" has meant "man," human rights have been rights for men only, and "persons" has meant "male persons." But for women this voyage is fraught with hazards in a way it is not for men. Our theories of moral development, if they are to be theories of human moral development, will have to acknowledge this fact.

If what I have said is correct, education will also have to take women's and men's differential moral experiences into account. This may mean, among other things, that we will have to adopt an approach to moral education which Jane Martin (1981) calls "gender sensitive," an approach which challenges the presumption that we can ignore gender in doing moral education.

CONCLUSION

In large part I have been engaged in what Adrienne Rich has called "the politics of asking women's questions" (1979, p. 17). I have tried to indicate the sorts of questions that we as women should ask of any ethics proposed in our name, and of any ethics it is proposed that we adopt.

My remarks have not been a defense of Noddings's theory nor a defense of the voices articulated in Gilligan's research. Indeed, they have been somewhat critical of both. However, it should be clear that my remarks represent a commitment to their enterprise—the enterprise of trying to describe how women themselves understand their own morality. We owe a great debt of gratitude to both Gilligan and Noddings for making that enterprise possible.

NOTES

1. It should be noted that what Baier calls "the teachability" is a more stringent requirement than the claim that morality must be learnable. This latter requirement would also satisfy the general presupposition that 'ought implies can', but I think Baier is correct to insist on the more stringent criterion.

2. This question was first posed by Kathryn Pynne Adelson in a public lecture at Carleton College in 1980.

3. This is not a direct quotation, but essentially the question Card asks.

4. It should be noted that Noddings does not formalize these prescriptions as rules or anything like rules. Indeed, she might well regard my minimal formalizing of these (loosely called) prescriptions as antithetical to the spirit of her work. Certainly both Gilligan and Noddings stress the need to avoid abstract principles and to attend

carefully to the particular situation in order to see what is to be done. Nevertheless, I think it not wholly misleading to consider these several prescriptions as part of Noddings's account of what it is to care for someone. Further, I am not wholly persuaded that the directive to attend to the context is helpful enough. But more on this later.

5. Noddings makes it clear that this prescription would arise only in a context in which it was expected that the relationship would continue over a long time. She also makes it clear that in following this prescription one would be acting in a supererogatory manner. I agree with her; my worry is that in the division of moral labor that has paralleled the sexual division of labor, women have generally been assigned the supererogatory moral labor as part of their role as women. Thus, for them, the supererogatory is not easily distinguishable from the obligatory.

6. Noddings's response was clarified in a public discussion at The Association for Moral Education Meetings in Toronto, November 1985. Certainly the first part of her answer is in her book. If my memory is correct, the second and third parts are the sort of answers she gave in public discussion.

7. In Canada, a woman is sexually assaulted every six minutes; and one woman in ten married or living with a man is so severely beaten by her partner as to require medical attention. In the United States, a woman is raped every three seconds; every 18 seconds a woman is beaten severely enough by her husband to require hospitalization (Morgan 1984). In the single Commonwealth of Massachusetts, every 22 days a woman is murdered by her husband or by a heterosexual lover (*Boston Globe* 1987). The statistics on rape and battery are generally conservative given the difficulty in estimating unreported incidents. These statistics do not include the sexual abuse of girls as children. Again, accurate figures are difficult to obtain, but responsible researchers estimate that somewhere between 10 to 25 percent of girls are victims of sexual abuse as children (Rush 1980).

8. For a reminder of our failure to consider the damage done to women by their oppression when we do research on women's caring for others, see Joan Ringelheim (1985).

REFERENCES

Atkinson, T. (1974). *Amazon Odyssey*. New York: Link Books.
Baier, A. (1985). What do women want in moral theory? *Nous* 19, (1): 53–63.
_____ . (1986). Trust and antitrust. *Ethics* 96: 231–260.
Baier, K. (1965). *The moral point of view*. Ithaca, NY: Cornell University Press.
Blum, L., Homiak, M., Housman, J., and Scheman, N. (1979). Altruism and women's oppression. In *Philosophy and women*, ed. M. Bishop and M. Weinzweig. Belmont, CA: Wadsworth.
Boston Globe. (1987). Critics fault police unit in Hub murder. *The Boston Globe*, June 29.
Card, C. (1985). Virtues and moral luck. Working paper series 1, Institute for Legal Studies, University of Wisconsin-Madison Law School.
Frye, M. (1983). *The politics of reality: Essays in feminist theory*. Trumansberg, NY: The Crossing Press.

Gilligan, C. (1982). *In a different voice: Psychological theory and women's development*. Cambridge, MA: Harvard University Press.

Goodman, E. (1982). Do gobetweens really smooth the path? *The London Free Press*, February 27.

Grimshaw, J. (1986). *Philosophy and feminine thinking*. Minneapolis, MN: University of Minnesota Press.

Martin, J. (1981). The ideal of the educated person. *Educational Theory* 31: 97–109.

Morgan, R. (1984). *Sisterhood is global*. Garden City, NY: Anchor Press/Doubleday.

Noddings, N. (1984). *Caring: A feminine approach to ethics and moral education*. Berkeley, CA: University of California Press.

Nunner-Winkler, G. (1984). Two moralities? A critical discussion of an ethic of care and responsibility versus an ethic of rights and justice. In *Morality, moral behavior and moral development*, ed. W. M. Kurtines and J. L. Gewirtz. New York: Wiley.

Rich, A. (1979). *Lies, secrets, and silence*. New York: Norton.

Ringelheim, J. (1985). Women and the Holocaust: A reconsideration of research. *Signs* 10: 741–761.

Rush, F. (1980). *The best kept secret: Sexual abuse of children*. Englewood Cliffs, NJ: Prentice Hall.

Part II

**EMPIRICAL STUDIES OF
THOSE WHO CARE**

6

Ways of Knowing, Learning, and Making Moral Choices

Nona Lyons

INTRODUCTION

When psychologists Blythe Clinchy and Claire Zimmerman (1975) first began to study how college-age women understood the nature of knowledge and came to construct their own truths instead of accepting without question the precepts of authority or their own gut reactions, they were guided by the work of William Perry (1970). College students, Perry argues, move during their undergraduate years from a dualistic understanding that knowledge can be cast as either right or wrong to a position of relativism, an understanding that all knowledge is constructed. In sketching these changes, Perry suggests that what is needed to achieve this epistemological revolution is a capacity for detachment, an ability to stand back from oneself in objectivity, to assess conflicting authorities and the relativism of one system of thought to another (Perry 1970, p. 35).

Most of the college women Clinchy and Zimmerman studied could match the positions and changes in thinking of Perry's Harvard men. But they did something else not predicted by Perry's model. While the women were able to act in detached objectivity, to see and respond to demands of external authorities, they also acted out of a need to understand the opinions, beliefs, and perspectives of other people. In brief, in order to understand others they seemed to step into, not back from, situations, to see and respond to others in their own particular situations and contexts. Later, Clinchy joined with Belenky, Goldberger, and Tarule (1986) to elaborate and verify these findings for a more diverse group of women.

Using a sample of 135 women, including women in city colleges as well as rural mothers coping under difficult, sometimes oppressive, situations, Belenky et al. (1986) confirmed the earlier findings of women's multiple

approaches to knowing, but expanded their theory to include five different epistemological perspectives. These categories range from "silence"
and "received knowledge," places where women look to others as
authorities, denying their own voices; through a "subjectivist" belief
which affirms their own personal ideas; to a belief in a more systematic,
"procedural knowing"; and, finally to a conception, similar to Perry's,
that all knowledge is contextual and constructed and that women are
"constructionists," capable also of "making theory."

In this work Belenky and her colleagues found that the metaphor of
"voice" captured accurately and most powerfully the way women came to
understand themselves as knowers, especially in "gaining a voice" or
finding one. Belenky and her colleagues found, too, a link between
women's ways of knowing, their ideas about themselves and questions of
value—about what is right and wrong, good and bad. Thus, in connecting
these ideas of self, morality, and epistemology, Belenky et al. expanded
on what Carol Gilligan (1977; 1982) first suggested and my work (Lyons
1981; 1982; 1983) confirmed, that is, that there is an intricate connection
between people's ideas of self and their ideas about morality.

This chapter takes up issues of morality, self, and approaches to knowing of adolescent high school girls. It examines in a clearly speculative
way how girls' ways of knowing are linked to the logic of their ideas of
self and morality by using two different kinds of data: (1) an examination
of typical constructions of moral conflicts reported by adolescent girls,
and (2) an examination of epistemological perspectives found in girls'
responses to a story completion task about different theories of how the
universe was formed. The recent research on women's ways of knowing
of Belenky et al. (1986) provides one context for this work, as does
research that first established an ethic of care (Gilligan 1977; 1982) and
more recent work on adolescent girls' ways of making moral choices
(Gilligan and Lyons 1985). In the first part of this chapter I present some
examples of adolescent girls' use of two orientations to morality, a
morality of justice and a morality of care (Gilligan 1977, 1982; Lyons
1982, 1983) and show how these orientations may be seen as ways of
knowing. Second, I present and discuss the story completion exercise and
indicate girls' different epistemological perspectives. Third, I address the
potential educational implications of this work, that is, of different approaches to learning implied in different ways of knowing. I conclude
with a discussion of how teachers in one high school, the Emma Willard
School, have thought about and used this research in their own teaching.
Here, ideas first revealed through research identifying an ethic of care,
help elaborate care and justice, suggesting new dimensions of both and
offering a program for future research.

THE CONNECTION BETWEEN IDEAS
OF SELF AND MORALITY

When Gilligan first challenged the field of moral psychology, she argued that moral psychology's traditional and singular focus on justice had obscured another dimension of people's moral concerns (Gilligan 1977, 1982). In addition to rights and fairness, the concerns of justice identified in Kohlberg's (1969, 1984) model of moral development, Gilligan suggested that other issues shape people's ways of framing moral conflict and choice: that is, concerns about interdependence, about maintaining the connections and attachments between individuals or assuring that someone not be excluded or hurt. Gilligan called this orientation to morality an ethic of care or response. Gilligan had identified this orientation to morality in part by studying women, whom, she found, focused more frequently than men on these issues of response and care in their moral decision-making.

My own work, the first systematic testing of Gilligan's hypotheses, analyzed people's use of the two moral orientations in describing their actual life conflicts and looked at the relationship between people's self-descriptions and the moral conflicts they described (Lyons 1981, 1982, 1983). Results revealed a complex pattern. Men and women used both justice and response (care) considerations in their reasoning about moral conflict; however, people were likely to focus predominantly on one orientation. Similarly, while men and women could focus on either orientation, women were more likely to focus on response considerations while men were more likely to focus on considerations of equality and fairness in relationships. In this analysis, I identified, too, the link between the ways individuals described themselves and their ways of thinking about moral choice.

The key issue in connecting self-description with moral orientation is the way individuals describe the relationships between people. Although most people, men and women, mention relationships in their self-descriptions, there are differences. People characterizing themselves as autonomous or 'separate' in their relations to others more frequently use considerations of justice and fairness in their moral decision-making; people describing themselves as interdependent or 'connected' in their relations to others more frequently use considerations of response or care. Thus, this work called attention to the significance of relationships, of the attachments between people, as the intricate link between a person's ideas of self and morality. The need then was to investigate and elaborate more specifically how relationships figured in people's changing understandings of self and their deliberations in moral choice.

THE EMMA WILLARD STUDY OF ADOLESCENT GIRLS

Our research in moral psychology, especially the discovery of women's moral concerns, attracted the attention of administrators at the Emma Willard School, an all girls high school in Troy, New York. Founded in 1814, Emma Willard is a school with a traditional concern about excellence in the education of women. Looking to current formulations in psychology to help them think about the education of girls in the 1980s, Emma Willard administrators were dismayed to find that in 1981 there was not very much research to help them understand girls' development or their learning. Like psychologist Joseph Adelson (1980), who at that time was also seeking to summarize recent research on adolescent girls, they concluded with a stark assessment: that "adolescent girls have just not been much studied" (Adelson 1980). It was then that Emma Willard officials asked Gilligan to help them think through the issue of the education of girls. In particular they wanted to know how girls thought about and made choices about their courses of study, their school counsellors, roommates, their future, and themselves. Thus, Gilligan and I, joined by other women researchers from Harvard, began a study of Emma Willard girls' ideas about choices, including as a central exploration their moral choices.

The idea that this would be an important study of adolescent girls and that theory from moral psychology could inform an understanding of adolescent girls' behavior intrigued the Emma Willard staff and they became eager students of this research. Discussions between faculty and researchers in formal workshops and in informal conversations took place over the four years of the project. These conversations, which focused on both issues of theory and practice, shaped new questions to be added to the study and raised issues about how staff intrepreted the behavior of their students as well as how they might modify their practices. Through open-ended interviews Emma Willard girls began to share their ideas about themselves, their life in school, their understandings of relationships, the moral conflicts they saw and dealt with in their lives, and how they envisioned their future. The project was designed to map aspects of girls' development and to examine and revise educational practices in one school setting.

Two Emma Willard high school students exemplify the predominant use of either justice or care reasoning found in the thinking of Emma Willard students who took part in this study (Gilligan and Lyons 1985; Gilligan, Lyons, and Hanmer, in preparation). The two students presented here are meant to represent a larger sample of people, male and female, who have similarly been found to use justice or care as a predominant pattern in making moral choices (Lyons 1982, 1983; Gilligan et al. 1982; Johnston 1985; Gilligan and Lyons 1985). Although it has also been found that there can be a third pattern in the use of justice and care reasoning, that is, an equal use of both justice and care considerations, here each is discussed separately for purposes of contrast. My intention is to identify and connect features of knowing to a person's characteristic use of justice or care reasoning in her moral decision-making.

A MORALITY OF JUSTICE AND A MORALITY OF CARE: WAYS OF KNOWING

Responding to an interview question asking them to tell about a moral conflict they faced, two adolescent girls, leaders in the organizations and affairs of their school, reveal situations that caused them conflict: situations they describe as moral conflicts. It happens that the conflicts they present pertain to their leadership duties. One girl, Jane, the editor of a school publication, begins by identifying a situation she faced when a member of her editorial staff failed to carry out her job. Describing the situation and her problem, Jane says:

I had a problem with a . . . girl whom I would tell her that I needed her to get something done and I would tell her two weeks ahead of time and then I would go re-mind her . . . and she would kind of act like I was nagging her about it. So I wouldn't say anything to her and, then, when I needed whatever she was supposed to have done, she hadn't done it. And this went on for about two months. It took me a long time . . . I felt like I really knew that I needed somebody else to be doing the job and, yet, I felt that whenever I would talk things over with her, she would say, "Yah, I really want to do it and I want to be able to help." It's like I kept feeling torn between should I get someone new and say you are fired, or should I just keep waiting. I guess I finally decided that I looked at things she was doing . . . wasn't really sure, partly I wasn't sure if I should be dealing with her or I should ask my faculty adviser to go speak to her so I wouldn't have to get involved. I finally decided that it was probably better if I talked to her, because it was really a problem between me and her and the faculty adviser wasn't involved.

Another student, Tracy, a proctor in one of the school's dormitories, responsible for some ten students in her hall, reveals a situation of conflict that occurred for her:

This year as a proctor, I am supposed to mark people off and at the beginning of the year, I was very concerned with really doing, being a straight arrow and doing a good job. And somebody once asked me, one of the three musketeers, one of my good friends, who I lived with, asked me if she could sleep through "Morning Reports" assembly which is never supposed to be done, because I am supposed to mark her off if she is there. And that was hard, because I was caught between choosing between a friend and what was right.

Asked to specify the conflict, Tracy goes on:

It was the difference between choosing, doing what the rule said, what the rules dic-tated and maintaining my friendship with this girl, at least as I saw it, to maintain my relationship with this girl.

While both girls hold positions of leadership and could have invoked the authority of their position to resolve the conflicts they report, they did not. Tracy, for example, could have told her friend, "No, you can't sleep in." Similarly, Jane could have said, "Have your assignment in by Friday or I will have to replace you." And while the conflicts they report could have been cast quite similarly—"I had a problem in doing my job"—they are cast with different emphases. Tracy exemplifies a justice focus and Jane a response one. Table 6.1 presents a comparison of the problems the girls saw, indicating in each student's own words how the problem was construed, the considerations each person brought to its resolution and to the evaluation of the resolution. While these differences may at first appear subtle, they are nonetheless identifiable.

The contrast between these students reveals different elements in priority. For the proctor the challenge of rule versus friendship is cast as an issue of hierarchy—the priority of her friendship versus her authority in maintaining the rules. For the editor the conflict is twofold, both wanting to honor the girl's desire to keep the job on the school journal, and, when she fails to do her assignments, of confronting her. Here it is not just that different kinds of conflict engage these young women, but each girl frames the conflict differently.

Examining more carefully the features of these situations we see certain patterns to each girl's thinking. For Jane, the editor, a hesitant questioning is her first response to the situation. Maybe she was being unreasonable, unclear. Maybe she hadn't "made it clear the things needed to be done." As she ponders what she actually considered in thinking through what to do, we see at work this same questioning, "I wanted to yell at her . . . but I just couldn't look at my situation as the most important." Seeing what else is going on in the girl's life, stepping into her situation and context, forces Jane to stop. Then by taking on the work of the other girl she comes to recognize, too, that she is hurting herself. There is no good solution in doing the work herself. Similarly, she recognizes that other people, in taking up the slack and doing added work, were finding it too much for them. Ultimately she decides she must decide for herself, confront the girl, and when she does, is amazed to discover that the girl is not upset to give up her job.

Categorizing aspects of Jane's thinking, several features can be identified. She

is tentative and questioning: she questions if she is right;

is context oriented: looks to see the other in her situation and context;

tests her reading of the conflict with those involved; seeks understanding of self and other;

uses dialogue with others to assess the problem and find a solution;

deliberates more about solving the problem than any other aspect of it.

Table 6.1

Analysis of Two Kinds of Moral Conflict: Considerations Used in the Construction of the Problem, the Resolution, and the Evaluation of the Resolution

Conflict 1: Jane, the Editor

1. I didn't really want to confront her and I knew I had to.

2. I didn't know if I was being un-reasonable in things I was asking her to do—maybe I didn't make it clear to her the things I needed [her] to do.

Resolution

1. Part of me wanted to yell at her—but when I would see her upset about things that were going on in her life or just other things that she was busy with, I couldn't just go and say, "You know, why aren't you doing this..." I just couldn't look at my situation, that this is the most important thing because I real-ized there were other things going on.

Conflict 2: Tracy, The Proctor

1. It was a difference between choosing what the rule said, what the rules dictated, and... maintaining my friendship with this girl.

Resolution

1. I considered that she knew my job. She knew what kind of pressure I was under and if she was going to sit there and pressure me, what kind of friend was she and if I said "No" to her over morning reports and she de-cided this was the end of our friendship, maybe we didn't have that much of a friendship.

Table 6.1 (continued)

<u>Resolution</u>

2. One of my decisions was taking on the work that she hadn't done and not really dealing with her...I guess I could have conceivably kept her on and her never really doing the work and...[but] I would end up feeling bad about it because I did.

3. I also talked to some other people about it on staff [asking] "What do you think?"...so I was passing it off like "Do you know why she isn't doing this?"

4. And everyone else was sort of doing her job and it was getting to be too much work for other people. I guess I had to decide, me decide.

<u>Evaluation</u> (<u>Was it the right thing to do?</u>)

1. Yeah. I think looking back on it I do. In some ways because I knew she really wanted to do it and in the beginning I felt bad. I could say "Yeah, she really does want to do it." But I feel now that it was the right thing because obviously

<u>Resolution</u>

2. I was at a point where I needed to assert my authority as a leader and she needed some limits set for her.

<u>Evaluation</u>

1. Sure, yeah, because it's important at the beginning of the year to draw, at least to start with, a hard line because then it makes it a lot easier to ease up later. And I didn't want to start easy and then to tighten up.

110

she wasn't upset by what happened in
the end. It was more upsetting when
there were problems going on.

2. ...At this point in time, I was at
the point that I needed to assert my
authority as a leader and she needed
some limits set for her, too,
because she was at the period where
she was testing me out to see what I
would do...because it was new in the
year. She had known me as somebody
who fooled around the year before, I
mean by being late to study hall and
not regarding the rules as a sacred
cow and saying "That is a stupid
rule and I am going to violate it
because I don't feel it has a lot of
merit," so she was testing me out to
see what kind of an authority figure
...I was going to be and I needed to
say to her, "Hey, you are not going
to be able to use our friendship as
a tool to push me around."

3. I realized that you can do what is
right and at the same time not sacrifice relationships. As my friends
have gotten older they have an
ability to do that, too...I believe
this is right and the world is going
to die unless this happens and she
believes something else very

111

Table 6.1 (continued)

Evaluation (Was it the right thing
to do?)

Evaluation

strongly and we are able to argue
about that. In fact, we are able to
fight a lot and still get along, and
our friendship still works. And
that can work. I have discovered
that you can do the "right" thing
and not sacrifice a relationship.

One might say in the end that Jane learns something about the girl and herself. It was more upsetting living the situation than confronting the person, a kind of psychological knowledge of the interactions between individuals.

Similarly, characterizing aspects of Tracy's thinking, several features are revealed. She:

is assertive and self-referencing;

is oriented to seeing the problem in terms of how it meets a standard she holds ("if she were going to pressure me, what kind of a friend was she . . . maybe we didn't have that much of a friendship");

seeks understanding of self by others ("She knew what kind of pressure I was under.");

casts the problem as if within a hierarchy ("choosing what the rule said or maintaining my friendship.");

fits the problem to a general situation ("I needed to assert my authority as a leader and she needed some limits set for her, too, . . . she was at the period where she was testing me out to see what I would do.");

deliberates more about how she evaluates her decision, that is, how she justifies her actions.

In the end Tracy learns something about friendship and herself, that you can keep to your standards, do the right thing, and still have a relationship. It is a balance the individual can achieve, a psychological knowledge of the self about relationships.

Table 6.2 summarizes the logic of two moral perspectives and Table 6.3 shows a related set of ideas. In particular I draw attention to the features of knowing and thinking evident in each orientation. While these summaries were prepared and developed from previous studies of people's use of justice and response of care reasoning as well as the Emma Willard study, it is useful here to see how a set of related ideas—of self, relationships, and ways of thinking—are interconnected to ideas about morality (Lyons 1982, 1983, 1985). It is important to restate, too, that most people—including the students presented here—show evidence of both kinds of considerations in their thinking about moral conflict. Yet it is the patterning of these responses so that one mode predominates, shaping the way issues are constructed and resolved, that is of interest.

Ways of Knowing: Another Perspective

The task was straightforward: Complete the story. It was presented to 73 Emma Willard students with these instructions:

Table 6.2
An Overview of the Central Moral Issues and Logic of Care and Justice in the Construction, Resolution, and Evaluation of the Resolution of Moral Dilemmas

MORALITY OF CARE/RESPONSE

A. In What Becomes a Moral Problem

A morality of "care" rests on an understanding of relationships that entails
response to another in their terms and
contexts. Therefore, what becomes a
moral problem has to do with relationships or the activities of care.

The conflicts of relationships are raised
as issues surrounding the potential
fractures between people, that is, with
the breaking--not of trusts or obliga-
tions--but the severing of ties between
people; or conversely, with restoring or
maintaining relationships.

The conflicts surrounding the activities
of care have to do with response itself,
that is, how to respond (or the capacity
or ability to respond) to another within
the particular situation one encounters:
how to promote the welfare or well-being
of another; or, to relieve their burdens,
hurt or suffering--physical or psychological. Included in this construction
can be particular concerns about care of
self, how to care for self especially in
considering care of others.

MORALITY OF JUSTICE/RIGHTS

A. In What Becomes a Moral Problem

A morality of justice as fairness rests
on an understanding of relationships as
reciprocity between separate individuals. Therefore, what becomes a
moral problem has to do with either:
mediating issues of conflicting claims
in the relationships between people; or
with how one is to decide conflicts or
how one can justify one's decision and
actions, considering fairness as a goal
between individuals.

The moral dilemmas of conflicting claims
have to do with the conflicts of obligation, duty or commitment stemming from
the different role-relationships one may
have, that is, between self and others,
self and society or to one's own values/
principles. The conflicts with respect
to how one is to decide come from the
need to have some impartial, objective
measure of choice that insures fairness
in arriving at a decision.

B. In the Resolution of Moral Conflict

In a morality of care resolutions to moral conflict are sought: (1) in restoring relationships or the connections between people; (2) in carrying through the activities of care, ensuring that good will come to others or that hurt/suffering will be stopped for others or oneself.

C. In the Evaluation of the Resolution

In the morality of care the evaluation of moral choice is made considering (1) whether relationships were restored/or maintained; (2) how things worked out or will work out; and in some instances there is only the acknowledgment that there is no way to know/to evaluate resolution. Whether relationships were restored can be measured in several ways: simply if everyone is happy, if people talk to one another, or if everyone is comfortable with the solution. If people talk and everyone agrees with the solution, one knows relationships are maintained.

B. In the Resolution of Moral Conflict

In a morality of justice resolutions to moral conflicts are sought considering (1) meeting one's obligations or commitments or performing one's duties; or, (2) in holding to or not violating one's standards, principles, especially fairness.

C. In the Evaluation of the Resolution

In a morality of justice, the evaluation of moral choice is made considering: (1) how the decision was justified, thought about; or (2) whether values, standards or principles were maintained, especially fairness.

How the decision was justified or thought about is an important measure to make of living up to one's obligations (duty or commitments) or of fairness; whether values, standards or principles were maintained is a measure of both the self's ability to live up to one's obligations or principles and a measure too of the standards used in decision-making.

Table 6.2 (continued)

How things work out is a measure of resolution in that in seeking what happens to people over time, one then knows if the resolution worked. This marker also carries the notion that <u>only</u> over time can one know results, that is, know in the sense of seeing what actually happens.

*Extracted from <u>A Manual for Coding Real-Life Dilemmas</u>, Lyons 1982.

116

Table 6.3
The Logic of Two Moral Perspectives: A Set of Related Ideas

	The Perspective of Response in Relationships	The Perspective of Rights in Relationships
Perspective toward others	Tries to see others in their own terms and contexts. Enter into their situation.	See others as one would like to be seen, in equality and reciprocity. Step back from situation for objectivity.
Conception of self-in-relation to others	Interdependent in relation to others.	Autonomous/equal/independent in relation to others.
Ideas and images of relationship	Attachment as given, interdependence of people; concern with responsiveness, isolation of people; relationships as webs.	Attachment through roles; obligation, duty; concern with equality and fairness in relationships; relationships as hierarchies.
Mode of thinking/knowing	Particularistic; contextual; suspended question posing; use of dialogue, judgment; goal is understanding; thinking and feeling held together.	Objective; generalizing; abstract; rule-seeking; goal is to critique; analyze; to answer question; to prove; thinking and feeling seen as needing to be separated.
Interpersonal ideas and processes	Interdependent; emphasis on discussion; listening; in order to understand others in own contexts.	Objective; role-related; in order to maintain fairness and equality in dealing with others.

117

The following situations are ones high school students sometimes face. For each situation, complete the story. Tell what the person is thinking and feeling and what they might do. Since these are stories there are no right or wrong ones.

One of the story situations given to the high school students included this short narrative:

The teacher has said that there were three theories of how the universe was formed. Sandy wondered: "How could there be three theories?"

The high school students wriggled in their seats, pondered how they might complete the stories and then wrote their own. These are the stories four different students wrote:

1. Only three? Why not hundreds. After all the Indians thought that at night a big basket was put over the world. That's how we got stars,the holes in the basket. But why weren't there more? There had to be. So many people think differently. Okay. So only three were acknowledged. Let's see if the teacher can explain them and then I'll hit her with a few more. Why can't there be more than three?
2. "I'm sure you are all wondering what these three theories are," said the teacher. "For homework, I want you to read Chapter Five. Chapter Five tells you all three theories and explains them. If you still have questions tomorrow, I'll be happy to answer them."
3. Sandy, of course, could only believe in one theory and felt upset that it could be wrong. She was scared at the idea of not being able to understand the universe. How was she supposed to understand herself?
4. The only one she knew of was about Adam and Eve. She decided to ask her teacher what the theories were. The teacher explained. She still believed the Bible. Sandy had learned about how the universe was formed in Sunday School and had been brought up with that idea. She didn't want to believe the chemistry and biology that helped form it. The universe is very peaceful and plain and the astrological facts made it complicated and boring. She didn't wish to think of it that way. She liked to be plain and peaceful.

In these responses it is possible to see another example of adolescent girls' approaches to knowing. In the narratives they write, the girls present the sense they make of the motives of human conduct, and the values and goals which they see underlying human action. And in the particular story task, considering multiple theories of the universe, it is possible to identify patterns in girls' thinking which suggest that a more rigorous examination of these findings across different high school populations is an important research agenda, especially for educators.

For what is striking about these story examples is not just that they contain different ideas about authority or imply different underlying stances toward the nature of knowledge, but that embedded within them is a view of the self. Students' ideas about knowledge seem connected to their ideas about the self: whether knowledge is thought of as fixed and given by authorities or whether it is multiple: and, whether one is questioning and comfortable in the face of the multiplicity of knowledge or threatened by it. There may be a right answer and someone can surely tell you. ("Chapter Five tells you all three theories.") There may be many answers, each with its own truth. ("Only three theories? Why not hundreds?") But changing ideas about the nature of the world, of knowledge can appear as changing ideas about one's self as well, and these can clearly be experienced as threatening to an individual ("She was scared at the idea . . . "). Understanding the universe is linked to understanding the self. And believing something—like the role of chemistry or biology in the construction of the world—may be something one can refuse to do, as one student wrote. It may be "more peaceful" that way. Student responses reveal the self is intricately implicated in ways of knowing, as it is in ways of valuing and making moral choices (Lyons 1981, 1983).

Examination of the range of student approaches to knowing identified in the story of the multiple theories of the universe reveals that the 73 students who participated in this exercise were at different positions in their ideas regarding multiple theories. These ranged from those students who wrote about one right answer (12 percent or nine students); or that some "authority knows," for example, the teacher, a book (22 percent or 16 students); to those who expected "diversity," multiple answers, insofar as they saw and expected that there might be multiple theories (8 percent or six students). But the largest number of students seemed through their stories to be what can be called "questioners" (44 percent or 32 students). This category included a range, from those who were just beginning to perceive that questions might be asked about existing forms of knowledge, to those who saw that their current formulations were different from those of other students, to those who saw clearly the possibility of multiple theories. Some students saw multiplicity but did not want to confront it or acknowledge it in their thinking. In these data there was no correlation with grade level. Some ten student responses were identified as "other," and need further elaboration.

A summary of the ideas of different epistemological perspectives or categories along with some characteristic features of the self is presented in Table 6.4.

Theoretical Issues and Educational Implications of the Story Completion Exercise

The work presented here, the story completion responses, is clearly only in its formative stages. It does, however, offer some initial insights to teachers and researchers. Students who answered these questions and wrote their stories sit in classes next to one another. Their diversity of views—a fact teachers always wrestle with—is here identified in its knowledge dimensions,

Table 6.4
Epistemological Categories of High School Students with Related Ideas About the Self

	Epistemological Perspective		Idea of Self
1.	There is one right answer.	1.	Self seems hidden/less accessible.
2.	Authority knows.	2.	Self seems hidden/less accessible.
3.	Questioning: multiplicity perceived.	3.	Self in transformation; may be frightened by what is glimpsed/perceived in what is or what can be known; knowledge may be rejected.
4.	Diversity expected.	4.	Self appears comfortable, even playful, in face of multiplicity.

suggesting that students may be at quite different but identifiable epistemological places. Although teachers have rarely had access to this kind of information, for researchers have not always addressed high school students, it seems important that the educational implications of these ideas be further developed not just as guides to teachers' understanding but also as ideas teachers may find useful in setting goals for student learning.

For example, if most students in a grade, class or school were in a questioning mode, that is, just beginning to perceive multiplicity, that would be most useful for teachers to know, if one goal were to aid students toward understanding the multiple and contextual nature of knowledge. Kitchener and King's work (Kitchener and Kitchener 1981; Kitchener 1983; King, Kitchener and Wood 1985) suggests that high school students as a whole share similar understandings about knowledge. But the research reported here indicates that a greater diversity may exist within a single class of students. Clearly it would be useful if teachers had a simple method, such as a set of story completion tasks, that they might use to identify the thinking of their students. Obviously there are diverse ways to interpret these data that we need to understand better. Psychologist Ellen Langer (1987) offers one perspective. Writing about how students learn, Langer emphasizes that her research indicates the power of student uncertainty as a special opportunity for learning. The danger of a teacher's helping behavior, for example, in providing a 'right answer' may be an impediment to student development.

Similarly, if teachers knew the kind of vulnerability of self in relation to knowing that students can experience, they might be able to respond to students in more useful and helpful ways. The data examined here, the stories of adolescent girls, indicate the vulnerability of students who confront the idea of multiplicity. On the basis of similar findings Perry (1970) posits special positions, like "retreat," that students find more comfortable in the face of multiplicity. Belenky et al.'s (1986) work suggests the special significance for adult women in development of finding a voice, of acknowledging oneself as a knower. Clearly the epistemological perspectives presented here need to be verified and elaborated for a range of students, male and female, before we can posit exact implications for teaching.

This work also suggests that there may be developmental aspects to, or changing understandings of, the nature of knowledge. For example, it seems possible that if a student once perceived that there might be multiplicity of views, she could not easily relinquish that understanding even if she wanted to. The question then is, is there a sequence to development in outline here? Do students move through these different perspectives sequentially as places in their development, or, do they constantly go through them, circling back as different areas or disciplines are encountered, a suggestion Perry (1970) makes. Belenky et al. (1986) do not confirm if their model is developmental. But the work of Kitchener and King (Kitchener and Kitchener 1981; Kitchener 1983; King et al. 1985) and Brabeck (1984) reveals an age-related developmental trend in changing ways of knowing among high school students.

It would also be interesting to compare this new model of epistemological perspectives of high school students with Belenky et al.'s (1986) work. A rough approximation has been suggested by Clinchy and Goldberger (1987) that lines up the "One Right Answer" and "Authority Knows" positions presented here with the "Received Knowers" of Belenky et al.'s model and the "Questioning Perceived" and "Multiplicity Expected" with Belenky's "Subjectivists," indicating that there may be more varied epistemologies among high school students than their model or Perry's indicates.

This work raises the issue, too, of the interaction between student and teacher and reminds us that learning takes place in relationships. The views of students presented here incorporate clear ideas about authority. While we do not know exactly how they translate these ideas and fit them with their own teachers, if they see their teachers as authorities, these student responses give some insights that are worthy of further inquiry, something we need to understand better.

IMPLICATIONS FROM THE EMMA WILLARD EXPERIENCE: A MODEL OF LEARNERS' INTERESTS AND GOALS

We know from the work at Emma Willard School that this research, in particular the identification of the two moral orientations in the thinking of

Emma Willard girls and the phenomenon of a focus or predominance in girls' thinking, is illuminating and useful to teachers in a number of ways. First it can help to account for and explain girls' behavior. Girls who value, for example, the maintenance of relationships, the welfare of their friends, the significance of principles, or all of these, act on them in their day-to-day life in the school.

The faculty adviser of Jane, the editor, for example, knew of her situation because she had asked the adviser for help. But the adviser had no idea how long the situation had gone on, nor, perhaps more importantly, that it had taken such a toll on Jane, in the work she took on and in the kind of thinking she carried out as she struggled to find a workable solution (See "Reflections of Emma Willard teachers," in Gilligan, Lyons, and Hanmer, in preparation).

Similarly, teachers seeing the two moral orientations as embodying two logics, now look at discipline issues differently. They recognize that girls may want to be involved in the school judiciary procedures for very different reasons—reasons that will shape their behavior: some to help prevent student troubles; others to have a chance to be in charge of the procedures that will guarantee fairness in deliberations. These views may be compatible. But they are subtly different, suggesting different values that in turn lead to different ways of interacting.

Probably the area of most significance to teachers comes in the ways teachers now think about the education of girls. Not only did Emma Willard faculty review and "balance" their curriculum to respond to the inclusion of women within it, that is, to guarantee that women were included (e.g., in the novels assigned in reading, in the examination in history of the social features of people's lives as well as the political features), but teachers became more attentive to their practices in support of student learning: in listening to questions students ask and in reflecting on their own responses; and in trying out diverse approaches, such as cooperative learning, in math classes and on the playing fields. Table 6.5 presents an hypothesized model of characteristic features of two approaches to learning implied in the two moral and self orientations, the justice and care modes with their related self-conceptions—the self as autonomous or separate and the self as interdependent or connected. (This terminology of a "connected" or "separate" knower is the one used by Belenky et al. (1986), adopted from my own work (Lyons 1981, 1982, 1983) and that of Gilligan (1977, 1982, 1986). Here the emphasis is on different features of the learner's goals and interests, which reflect different approaches to learning.

While the two approaches to learning are thought of as clearly complementary although significantly different, understanding and articulating these differences is an important agenda for the future. Most schools tend to foster rule-oriented, rational, abstract thinking, whether in math and science or history and social studies: less attention is given to features we

Table 6.5
Learners and Learning Contexts: The Relationship of Mode of Self to Learner's Interests, Goals and Mode of Thinking (Adapted from Belenky et al. (1986), Bruner (1986), Gilligan (1982), Lyons (1982, 1985))

Mode of Self	Learner's interests and goals	Learner as thinker and knower
Autonomous (separate in relation to others)	To question; to prove; to find answers to questions: to solve problems To convince by argument; logic Know how to know truth	Analytical; procedural; truth seeking; rule-seeking and using Test for truth: consistency; logic; reasoned hypothesis Transcend time and space and particulars; imagination: to see before proving; thought and feeling held apart
Interdependent (in relation to others)	To question; to find understanding of situations, people, and their contexts; narrative-seeking; to convince by motives, particulars of lives.	Tentative and questioning; judgment suspended; fact gathering; synthesizer Test for truth; believability; concern for understanding of human motivation; intention Imagination used to enter into situations, contexts; locate in time and place. Thought and feeling held together.

identify here as associated with a response of a "connected" learner. Emma Willard teachers, for example, found themselves thinking about student hesitancy and questioning in a different way once they had some familiarity with the two orientations. One new Emma Willard teacher of history, for example, shared an incident with colleagues which he at first found perplexing. He was nearing the end of a class in which he had been emphasizing how the American political system worked in one presidential election in which a deal was struck between Northern and Southern Democrats and Republicans. One girl raised her hand to ask what grounds the people involved had to trust one another. The teacher, feeling as if the question came from "left field" since it had nothing to do with a systems approach he was emphasizing, was puzzled at his failure to be clear. But in sharing this situation with colleagues he was offered a different interpretation. The girl was more interested as a learner in understanding the motives of those involved. She heard the event as a narrative, a story of an encounter in the relationships between individuals. The logic she sought was not the logic of a system. Rather she sought the logic of understanding, what Bruner calls "believability" (Bruner 1986). Unlike the teacher who sought to transcend time, she was rooted in it, in the particulars of the situation, and in the relationships between people. It is this approach to learning with its different concerns and interests that educators need to understand better and listen for. They also need to make opportunities for this voice to be expressed and heard. If this is a mode of learning more frequently found in the thinking of girls—although we know it is available to both sexes—we need to be attentive to that. Adolescent girls remind us of the centrality of Piaget's (1932/1965) insight, that apart from our relations to other people, there can be no moral necessity and let us understand how morality, mind, self, and relationships are intricately linked in everyday ways of knowing and learning.

ACKNOWLEDGMENTS

Research reported here was made possible by the generosity of the Geraldine R. Dodge Foundation who supported the Emma Willard School Study. I wish to thank Blythe Clinchy, Nancy Goldberger, and Monica Taylor, who kindly read drafts of this paper.

REFERENCES

Adelson, J., ed. (1980). *Handbook of adolescent psychology*. New York: John Wiley and Sons.
Belenky, M., Clinchy, B., Goldberger, N., and Tarule, J. (1986). *Women's ways of knowing*. New York: Basic Books.

Brabeck, M. (1984). Longitudinal studies of intellectual development during adulthood: Theoretical and research models. *Journal of Research and Development in Education* 17 (3):12–27.

Bruner, J. (1986). *Adult minds, possible words*. Cambridge, MA: Harvard University Press.

Clinchy, B., and Goldberger, N. (1987). Personal communication.

Clinchy, B. and Zimmerman, C. (1975). Growing up intellectually. Issues for college women. (Working Papers in Progress, No. 19). Wellesley, MA: Wellesley College, The Stone Center.

Gilligan, C. (1986). Exit-voice dilemmas in adolescent development. In *Development, democracy and the art of trespassing: Essays in honor of Albert O. Horschman*, ed. A. Foxley, M. McPherson, and G. O'Donnell. Notre Dame, IN: University of Notre Dame Press.

———. (1982). *In a different voice: Psychological theory and women's development*. Cambridge, MA: Harvard University Press.

———. (1977). In a different voice: Women's conceptions of self and morality. *Harvard Educational Review* 47: 481–517.

Gilligan, C., Langdale, C., Lyons, N., and Murphy, J. M. (1982). The contribution of women's thought to developmental theory. Final Report to the National Institute of Education. Cambridge, MA: Harvard University.

Gilligan, C., and Lyons, N. (1985). Listening to voices we have not heard. Report to the New York State Department of Education on the Emma Willard Study. Cambridge, MA: Harvard University.

Gilligan, C., Lyons, N., and Hanmer, T., eds. (In preparation). Making connections: Essays on the relational world of adolescent girls at Emma Willard school.

Johnston, D. K. (1985). Two moral orientations—two problem-solving strategies: Adolescents' solutions to dilemmas in fables. Ph.D. diss., Harvard Graduate School of Education.

King, P. M., Kitchener, K. S., and Wood, P. K. (1985). The development of intellect and character. A longitudinal-sequential study of intellectual and moral development in young adults. *Moral Education Forum* 10 (1): 1–13.

Kitchener, K. S. (1983). Cognition, metacognition and epistemic cognition: A three level model of cognitive processing. *Human Development* 26: 222–232.

Kitchener, K. S. and Kitchener, R. F. (1981). The development of natural rationality: Can formal operations account for it? In *Social development in youth: Structure and content*, ed. J. A. Meacham, and N. R. Santelli. Basel: S. Karger.

Kohlberg, L. (1969). Stage and sequence: The cognitive developmental approach to socialization. In *Handbook of socialization theory and research*, ed. D. Goslin. Chicago: Rand McNally.

———. (1984). *The psychology of moral development*. San Francisco: Harper and Row.

Langer, E. (1987). How students learn: On teaching and learning. *Journal of the Harvard-Danforth Center*. Harvard University.

Lyons, N. (1985). Visions and competencies: Men and women as decision-makers and conflict negotiators. Paper presented at American Educational Research Association, Boston.

_____ . (1983). Two perspectives: On self, relationships and morality. *Harvard Educational Review* 53:125–145.

_____ . (1982) Conceptions of self and morality and modes of moral choice. Ed.D. diss., Harvard University.

_____ . (1981). Manual for coding responses to the question: How would you describe yourself to yourself? Unpublished manuscript, Harvard Graduate School of Education.

Perry, W. (1970). *Forms of intellectual and ethical development in the college years.* New York: Holt, Rinehart and Winston.

Piaget, J. (1932/1965). *The moral judgement of the child.* New York: The Free Press.

7

Gender Differences in Empathy and Prosocial Moral Reasoning: Empirical Investigations

Nancy Eisenberg, Richard Fabes, and Cindy Shea

The notion that women are more caring, sympathetic, nurturant, and other-oriented than are men is pervasive (e.g., Block 1973; Parsons and Bales 1955; Shields 1987) and has received much attention from social and behavioral scientists in the last decade. This focus on gender differences in caring and sympathetic responses is due in part to the work of Carol Gilligan (e.g., 1977, 1982). Gilligan has argued that females and males, due to differential socialization, tend to develop two different approaches to morality: an ethic of caring and responsibility for females and an ethic of justice and rights for males. The ethic of care and responsibility develops from the individual's feelings of interconnectedness with others; the ethic of justice and rights is an expression of autonomy and the "individual self."

Specifically, the morality of care (the morality more often associated with women) "rests on an understanding of relationships as response to another in their terms" (Lyons 1983, p. 136). This focus on response to another directs attention to others and to the issue of how to act responsively. Thus, if Gilligan is correct, females, in comparison to males, would be expected to be more other-oriented in their moral judgments and more sympathetic to the plight or concerns of others. Moreover, we would expect parents and other socializers to differentially socialize children in ways that would encourage a stronger focus on others and their needs among girls than boys.

In this chapter we examine several notions relevant to the issue of gender differences in other-oriented moral reasoning and emotional responding.

The work described in this chapter was supported by current grants to the first author from the National Science Foundation (BNS-8509223 and BNS-8807717) and the National Institute of Child Health and Development (K04 HD00717), as well as prior grants from the National Institute for Mental Health and Arizona State University.

To accomplish this goal we first review the literature on gender differences in emotional responsivity and an other-orientation, and how these relate to differential socialization practices experienced by each sex. In later sections we briefly review the literature pertaining to gender differences in sympathy/empathy and moral reasoning and then present some of our own data concerning these issues.

GENDER DIFFERENCES IN EMOTIONAL RESPONSIVENESS

The belief that females are more emotionally responsive than males is one of the most common findings in research on gender-roles and gender-role stereotyping (e.g., Allen and Haccoun 1976; Brody 1985; Maccoby and Jacklin 1974). Even preschool children possess pronounced stereotypes about gender differences in emotionality and their stereotypes have been found to be similar to those held by adults (i.e., femaleness is negatively associated with anger and positively associated with happiness, sadness, and sometimes fear; Birnbaum and Chemelski 1984; Birnbaum, Nosanchuk, and Croll 1980; Brody 1985). Whether or not these perceived differences are based upon true differences between the sexes is still uncertain. However, numerous researchers have found differences in the emotional behavior of men and women. For example, researchers have established that females generally are superior to males in their abilities to decode (judge) and encode (express) nonverbal expressions of emotions (see Brody 1985; Hall 1978).

Moreover, the hypothesis that emotionality may differ for males and females is implicit in many theories of emotional development (e.g., Buck 1983; Chodorow 1978; Freud 1925/1950; Izard 1977; Kemper 1978). This is true for both biologically- and socially-based theories. Indeed, Hoffman (1977) noted that there appear to be no theories that contradict the stereotypes concerning gender differences in emotional responsiveness.

Although many biologically based theories of emotional development provide a basis for expecting gender differences (e.g., Izard 1977; Plutchik 1980), the available data do not support the notion that any differential emotional development for the two sexes can easily be accounted for by biological concomitants of emotion (Brody 1985). For example, gender differences in emotion-related biological processes (cerebral lateralization, neurochemical or hormonal substrates) are not well documented and their significance is uncertain when they are documented (e.g., Bryden 1979; Reinisch and Karow 1977; also see Huston 1983, for a recent review).

Social-cognitive theories of emotional development generally emphasize the importance of the social context for emotional development (e.g., Kemper 1978; Lazarus 1982; Lewis and Michalson 1983). From this perspective differential emotional development for the two sexes could occur because parents (and other social agents) socialize and relate to boys and girls differently. As a result, males and females are exposed to qualitatively different affective exchanges with caretakers (Chodorow 1978; Gilligan

1982; Parson and Bales 1955). For example, Parsons and Bales (1955) attributed differences in male and female emotionality to variations in traditional roles. In their view men are socialized to assume an instrumental role (characterized by tasks needed for the family and society to function) whereas females are socialized to assume an expressive role (characterized by tasks needed to facilitate interpersonal harmony in the family). To fulfill their respective roles females, but not males, are socialized to be nurturant, expressive, and affectionate.

Given the theoretical and stereotypic basis for predicting differences in emotionality between the sexes, we now examine the literature pertaining to the socialization of emotional behavior in boys and girls. Then we examine gender differences in the development of empathy and how differential socialization practices for boys and girls may be related to differences in empathic responsiveness.

GENDER DIFFERENCES IN THE SOCIALIZATION OF EMOTION

There is a growing body of literature consistent with the view that parents interact with girls and boys in ways that may differentially influence their emotional reactivity and other-orientation. For example, adults' perceptions of children's emotion-related behaviors vary according to the gender of the child. Condry and Condry (1976) found that the ratings made by adult males and females of an infant's emotional response varied according to whether they thought they were observing a boy or a girl. Across different situations, boys were rated as displaying more pleasure and less fear than were girls. Boys' crying was more likely to be perceived as anger whereas girls' crying was attributed to fear. Similarly, Wiesenfeld, Whitman, and Malatesta (1984) found that crying female infants were perceived as more distressed and more in need of being picked up than were crying male infants. Moreover, parents tend to perceive girls as more fragile and fearful than boys and worry more about daughters' than sons' well-being (Fagot 1981; Huston 1983).

Thus, adults' stereotypes about gender differences in emotionality influence their assessment of children's actual emotional behavior. It is possible that parents transmit these stereotypes explicitly or implicitly to children by selectively reinforcing only those emotional behaviors that they feel are sex-appropriate (Birnbaum et al. 1980).

Other researchers have examined whether parents actually respond differently to children's emotions depending upon the child's sex. Block (1973) found that parents reported greater insistence on the control of feelings and their expression for their sons, whereas they tended to emphasize maintenance of close emotional relationships, verbal discussion of emotions, and physical displays of affection for their daughters. Block (1973) also found that parents encouraged their sons to be aggressive but unemotional, and their daughters to be emotional but unaggressive. Malatesta and Haviland (1982) found that mothers exhibited a significantly greater tendency to respond to the smiles of infant males than to the smiles of infant females. In addition, mothers were found to match more of their sons' than their daughters' facial expressions.

Furthermore, parents may talk about emotions in quantitatively and qualitatively different ways depending upon whether their child is a boy or a girl. Grief and her colleagues found that parents generally used more affective words when telling stories to their girls than to their boys; however, they also tended to emphasize anger more frequently for sons than for daughters (Grief 1984; Grief, Alvarez, and Ulman 1981). Moss (1974) also found that parents used more affective terms when addressing girls than boys. Dunn, Bretherton, and Munn (1987) found that mothers encouraged more communication about feelings by girls than by boys as early as 18 months of age. By 24 months, mothers of girls were more likely to initiate conversations about feeling states than were mothers of boys. Moreover, by 24 months the girls themselves were more likely to talk about feeling states than were the boys.

Although inconsistencies exist, the aforementioned data provide support for the idea that parents treat their boys and girls differently in regard to their emotionality. These studies also suggest that girls (relative to boys) are more likely to be encouraged to develop skills that relate to empathic responsiveness such as emotional expressiveness (particularly in regard to feelings of affection and sadness, but not anger and aggression) and emotional sensitivity (i.e., decoding others' emotional cues, particularly within interpersonal contexts).

GENDER DIFFERENCES IN EMPATHY

Prior Research: Gender Differences

The data reviewed to this point provide a basis for expecting gender differences in empathy and related capacities. Block (1976) and Maccoby and Jacklin (1974) reviewed the empirical literature in empathy and concluded that there was no evidence of gender differences. These reviewers, however, used a broad definition of empathy and did not differentiate among various related capacities (e.g., role-taking, social sensitivity, vicarious responding, etc.). Moreover, they compared studies in which empathy was assessed in a number of different ways. Thus, it is not surprising that these reviewers failed to find consistent gender differences across studies.

In another review, Hoffman (1977) differentiated between studies in which empathy was defined as an emotional response and those in which empathy was defined as role-taking or social sensitivity. Hoffman (1977) concluded that there was ample evidence to support the conclusion that girls are more affectively empathic than boys. However, most of the data Hoffman reviewed were obtained from studies that used a picture-story measure of empathy (i.e., a measure in which children hear stories about others in emotionally evocative situations and then are asked how they themselves feel). Drawing such a conclusion on the basis of a single measure of empathy may be misleading. For example, Lennon, Eisenberg, and Carroll (1983) found that children's scores on the picture-story measure of empathy were significantly higher when the experimenter was the same sex as the child. Because female experimenters have been used in more research on children's empathy, the higher scores of girls may be a function of their responsiveness to a same-sex experimenter. Thus, the validity of picture-story measures is questionable in regard to identifying gender differences in empathy (see Eisenberg and Lennon 1983).

More recently, Eisenberg and Lennon (1983; Lennon and Eisenberg 1987) reviewed the data regarding gender differences in affective empathy and found they varied as a function of the method used to assess empathy. There were considerable differences favoring females for self-report measures of empathy, especially questionnaire indexes. However, no gender differences were found when the measure of empathy was either physiological or unobtrusive observations of nonverbal behavior.

One interpretation of the aforementioned finding is that the gender differences for some indexes were due to social demand characteristics and personal presentational biases. When demand characteristics were high (i.e., it was clear what was being assessed) and subjects had conscious control over their responses (i.e., self-report indexes were used), gender differences were present. When demand characteristics were subtle but self-report indexes were used, gender differences were somewhat smaller (albeit significant). When demand characteristics were subtle *and* subjects were unlikely to exercise much conscious control over their responding (i.e., physiological indexes), no gender differences were found. Thus, it appears that the differences in findings across measures of empathy are due to the tendency of people to report reactions consistent with gender stereotypes when the stereotypes are salient and they can easily control their responses (i.e., as with self-report indexes). People may act in this manner to project a socially desirable image to others or to themselves.

An alternative explanation for the pattern of findings is that the different measures of empathy assess different types of emotional reactions. For example, self-report measures may more accurately differentiate between empathy/sympathy and personal distress (self-focused feelings of anxiety or discomfort in reaction to another's emotional state or condition) than do physiological and facial measures. Precisely worded self-report measures may also tap empathy and sympathy more directly than do physiological or facial indexes. However, it is still unclear which types of emotional responses tend to be assessed by the different measures of empathy (Lennon and Eisenberg 1987).

Prior Research: Gender Differences in the Socialization of Empathy

Although the data reviewed previously support the assertion that there is a link between socialization experiences and differential empathic responsiveness for boys and girls, only a few investigators actually have examined this relation. Feshbach (1975) found that empathy in girls was related to positive mother-daughter interactions whereas for boys (but not daughters) empathy was inversely related to fathers' encouragement of competition. In another investigation, Barnett, Howard, King, and Dino (1980) found a positive relation between empathy and gender-role stereotypic patterns of parents' empathy. Barnett et al. suggested that when the mother is considerably more empathic than the father, empathy may be identified as distinctly gender appropriate for females, thereby enhancing its development in girls. No relations, however, were found for boys' empathy scores and the empathy scores for either parent.

These data support Feshbach's (1982) suggestion that empathy in girls may be associated with maternal antecedents that are likely to foster prosocial behavior and a positive self-image. Specifically, Feshbach suggested that empathy in girls is positively associated with maternal tolerance, affection, and permissiveness, and negatively associated with conflict, rejection, punishment, and excessive control. These patterns were not found for boys or for father-daughter relations.

In our own research (Fabes et al. 1988), we have found that mothers' attitudes toward their children's emotional behavior were differentially related to their son's or daughter's emotional responsiveness to another's distress. Mothers who were relatively restrictive regarding their sons' emotional expressivity in situations in which the expression of emotion could be considered inappropriate (e.g., because it would hurt another's feelings) had boys who were relatively unexpressive facially but exhibited evidence of an outward focus (i.e., heart rate deceleration) in response to another's distress. For girls, fewer relations existed. Girls whose mothers were relatively controlling of their emotional reactions tended to show less facial sympathy in response to another's distress than did girls whose mothers had less controlling attitudes. Thus, mothers who reported being relatively restrictive with regard to children's inappropriate emotional expressions generally had children who were less overtly expressive but may have been more internally responsive (sympathetic) to others' needs (especially for boys).

The failure to find as many significant relations for girls as boys may be because of the social desirability of girls' being sympathetic; girls may be socialized to be more sympathetic than are boys regardless of the parents' general attitudes toward children's emotional responsiveness. This finding is in line with the hypothesizing of Eisenberg and Mussen (1978). They found significant positive relations between offspring's empathy and maternal affection, egalitarianism, nonrestrictiveness, and nonpunitiveness for sons but not for daughters, and suggested that the lack of relations for girls may have been due to a ceiling effect for the girls' empathy scores.

Empirical Findings from Our Laboratory

Because of the aforementioned potential problems with self-report indexes of empathy and the resulting ambiguity in the body of empirical work concerning empathy and sympathy, we have recently used multiple methods in our studies of vicariously induced emotional reactions. Specifically, we have used physiological responsivity (heart rate; subsequently referred to as HR) and facial reactions, as well as self-report indexes of responsivity (i.e., self-report of reactions in an experimental study and questionnaire indexes of the trait of empathy). In addition, we have attempted to differentiate, conceptually and empirically in our studies, between sympathy (other-oriented feelings of concern or sorrow) and personal distress (self-focused vicariously induced anxiety, discomfort, distress, etc.). In this research we have examined gender differences in vicarious responding, as well as other issues of interest.

We now briefly review findings from four studies relevant to the issue of gender differences in sympathy, empathy, and personal distress. Facial and physiological findings are emphasized, although we do discuss some of our findings on self-report indexes.

Facial Indexes. In all four studies, we included facial indexes of sympathy and personal distress. In general, we have not found marked evidence of gender differences; however, whenever a difference has been found, it favors females.

In the first study, 4 to 5 year olds observed two films (approximately 9 weeks apart) in which other children were injured and were depicted as distressed and crying. Children's sad/concerned and anxious/distressed facial reactions were taped unobtrusively while they were viewing the emotion-eliciting sections of the films. Overall, there were no differences in the facial reactions of boys and girls, although sad/concerned expressions increased in frequency with age for girls but not boys (Eisenberg, Mc-Creath, and Ahn 1988).

In another study involving 4 to 5 year olds and second graders, the children viewed film clips chosen to elicit either distress (anxiety: the children viewed children frightened in a thunder storm), or empathic sadness and sympathy (the children viewed a film of a child who was overtly sad because her pet died and a film of a child with spina bifida attempting to walk during therapy). Girls exhibited more sad facial reactions while viewing the film about the child with spina bifida; moreover, such displays decreased with age for boys but not girls (Eisenberg, Fabes, Bustamante, Mathy, Miller, and Lindholm 1988).

In the remaining two studies, the participants were elementary-school children and adults (college students). In the first study participants discussed prior experiences in which they had felt either concerned about their own welfare (a type of distress akin to personal distress) or concerned about another's welfare (i.e., engaged in a sympathy induction). Their facial expressions were monitored unbeknownst to the subjects (they were informed afterwards and their consent to use the tape was obtained). In this study female subjects exhibited significantly more concerned attention (i.e., sympathy) than did the males during the sympathy induction. The sexes did not differ in displays of distress or sadness in either induction (Eisenberg et al., in press).

In the last study, second and fifth graders and college students viewed a purported pilot local news show about a family who was in a car accident. The family was filmed in a local hospital and the mother discussed the problems that her son and daughter were having with regard to therapy and missing school (the children were shown bandaged and in bed). Males tended to exhibit less facial distress (i.e., anxiety) than did females while viewing the film ($p < .08$); moreover, facial distress decreased from second to fifth grade for males but not females. Males and females did not differ significantly in facial displays of sadness or concern.

In summary, our data on facial indexes of vicarious responding are consistent with the view that females are somewhat, but not markedly, more likely to exhibit personal distress and sympathy. In addition, it appears that such displays of negative emotion decrease somewhat with age for males, and that any gender differences in facial indexes of empathy and related reactions may increase somewhat in the school years. However, our findings were not strong or consistent; therefore, it would be inaccurate to conclude that we obtained strong evidence of gender differences. The rather weak findings, particularly in our earliest studies, may have been due to our failure to adequately differentiate among the various facial expresssions. In our more recent studies, our facial coding schemes have become progressively more refined and sophisticated. In addition, it is unclear whether the gender differences obtained in our research were due to real differences between males and females in emotional reactions or were due to a gender difference in the tendency to inhibit or mask facial displays of emotion (with males displaying less negative emotion with age; see Shennum and Bugental 1982).

Physiological Indexes. It is difficult to examine gender differences in vicarious emotional responding with HR because males and females may differ in HR at certain ages (if one sex is more physically fit than the other). However, there do not seem to be strong gender differences in HR in childhood; thus, our data from children are at least suggestive.

Thus far, we have used HR in three studies of vicarious responding (the last three studies described previously). In none of these studies have we obtained clear evidence of a gender difference in physiological responsivity. There were some gender differences in regard to the relation of HR to other indexes of empathy/sympathetic/personal distress for the preschoolers in the study in which they viewed three films; however, no clear or strong pattern emerged. Moreover, in the induction study, although females exhibited higher HR than males while engaged in the sympathy and distress inductions, this difference may have been due to differences in the physical conditioning of the two sexes (e.g., perhaps because of participation in sports). In brief, at this time our HR data do not indicate that there are clear differences in males' and females' vicarious emotional responding.

Self-report Data. Consistent with prior research (Eisenberg and Lennon 1983; Lennon and Eisenberg 1987), we frequently have obtained gender differences in males' and females' self-reports of sympathy and personal distress (or related responses). These differences seem to increase somewhat with age. In our studies with young children we find relatively few gender differences in self-reports of vicarious emotional responses, although in the study involving preschoolers and second graders, girls reported more fear and less happiness than did boys in reaction to the distressing film (Eisenberg, Fabes, et al. 1988). However, gender differences are more evident in our studies involving school-aged children and adults. For example, in the induction study, girls reported marginally more distress in the sympathy induction and significantly more distress and less happiness in the distress induction. In addition, there was a marginally significant tendency for reports of concern in the sympathy induction to increase with age for girls but not boys. Among adults, women reported more distress in both inductions than did men, and tended ($p < .11$) to report more sympathy induction. In summary, in this study females reported more distress and somewhat more concern than did males (Eisenberg, Schaller, et al., in press).

Similarly, in the study about the family in the hospital there was a marginally significant tendency for report of sympathetic reactions to the family to increase with age for girls but not boys. In addition, there was a marginally significant tendency for girls to report more distress than boys. Among adults, women reported significantly higher levels of sympathy and general negative mood and marginally more distress. As in the induction study, there was some evidence of gender differences in the report of males and females, with the differences tending to be clearer among adults (although differences between the self reports of adults and children could not be directly compared because the adjective lists used to obtain self-reports differed somewhat for the adults and children).

Summary

Based on the extant empirical data, it is not clear whether there are gender differences in empathy, sympathy, and personal distress. Females tend to report more of these emotional responses but they do not differ markedly from males in nonverbal and physiological reactions. The differences that do occur in nonverbal indexes favor females, although it is possible that males simply mask or inhibit their sympathetic and empathic reactions more than females. Given the lack of differences in the physiological data as well as the nonverbal and self-report data indicating more responsivity by females, we hypothesize that males and females do not differ significantly in their tendencies to react emotionally to others' emotional states (i.e., in empathy), but do differ somewhat in how they cognitively process and interpret their own vicarious emotional reactions. Females may be less likely than males to defend against experiencing such emotional reactions and may be more likely than males to attribute their reactions to sympathetic concerns.

GENDER DIFFERENCES IN MORAL REASONING

Prior Research Findings

The issue of gender differences in moral reasoning has been hotly debated (e.g., Baumrind 1986; Colby and Damon 1983; Gilligan 1982; Walker 1984). Because of the focus on this topic in other chapters in this volume, we will merely summarize the content and status of this debate.

Gilligan (1979, 1982) has argued that Kohlberg's (Colby and Kohlberg 1987; Kohlberg 1976) theory of moral judgment centers around the concepts of rights and justice and, consequently, a quest toward greater independence and individuality. She further suggests that these personal qualities are defined as desirable in our society for males but not females. Thus, Kohlberg's highest stages—stages that stress individuality and autonomy of moral standards—seem incompatible with society's emphasis on the desirability of nurturance and interconnectedness for females. In Gilligan's view, women are not less morally mature than are men; rather, they strive for qualitatively different objectives in their quest toward moral maturity. Specifically, Gilligan proposes that there are two different systems of morality, one more applicable to males' moral development (in that it revolves around an ethic of rights and justice) and one more applicable to that of females (in that it is an ethic of caring and responsibility).

On a more concrete level, Gilligan has hypothesized that (1) males score higher on Kohlberg's scheme of moral judgment because it focuses on rights and justice, and (2) women use more reasoning pertaining to a care orientation whereas men use more pertaining to a rights orientation. With regard to the first issue, according to recent reviews and papers, males and females do not differ markedly in their reasoning on Kohlberg's moral dilemmas, (see Baumrind 1986; Brabeck 1983; Rest 1979; Walker 1984). With regard to the second issue—that of relative use of a care orientation—the data are limited. According to preliminary work, however, females seem more likely than males to verbalize care-related concerns (see Lyons 1983). For example, Gibbs, Arnold, and Burkhart (1984) found that women expressed more empathic role-taking justifications in their reasoning about Kohlberg dilemmas. Similarly, Gilligan and Attanucci (1988) found that females (in samples of adolescents and adults) used a care orientation more than did males whereas males used a justice focus more than did females when talking about real-life moral conflicts and choices. However, using similar procedures for a sample of children and their parents, Walker (1987) did not replicate the findings of Gilligan and Attanucci. Thus, the issue of gender difference in moral orientation is far from resolved. (See also the chapter by Bebeau and Brabeck in this volume for additional discussion.)

Empirical Findings on Prosocial Moral Judgment

As we discussed previously, in Kohlberg's dilemmas issues related to caring and prosocial concerns are not central; rather, the focus is on justice, rights, and prohibition-related issues (i.e., laws, rules, the dictates of authorities, formal obligations). Moreover, in the real-life moral dilemmas used in some studies (e.g., Gilligan and Attanucci 1988; Walker 1987), issues related to justice, rights, care, or other moral or social conventional concerns all might be central, so it is difficult to examine relative use of care-related reasoning (because care-related issues are less relevant to some moral dilemmas than others). In contrast, Eisenberg's prosocial moral reasoning dilemmas focus on prosocial issues per se—the conflict between self-interest and the needs of others. Thus, research on the development of prosocial moral reasoning is a useful vehicle for examining moral judgments about dilemmas in which caring and responsibility for others are central themes.

Moreover, nearly all of the literature on gender differences in moral reasoning about caring dilemmas has been conducted with adolescents and adults rather than children. As a result, it is difficult to determine the age at which any gender difference in an other-oriented focus with regard to prosocial dilemmas might develop. If such gender differences are due to socialization, as is hypothesized by Gilligan (1982) and others, one would expect few gender differences in the moral reasoning of young children (Baumrind 1986). Rather, gender differences in other-oriented modes of reasoning would be expected to emerge sometime in childhood because there is some evidence of such a difference by mid-adolescence and early adulthood (Gilligan and Attanucci 1988; Lyons 1983).

The coding system for scoring prosocial moral judgment contains some categories of reasoning that specifically tap other-oriented concerns. In initial research on prosocial moral reasoning, Eisenberg-Berg (1979a) factor-analyzed children's and adolescents' scores on the various coding categories and found that one of the factors included several categories that seemed to reflect an other-oriented perspective. Categories that loaded on this factor at .35 or higher were concern with others' physical and material need, concern with others' psychological needs, reference to and concern with humanness, sympathetic orientation, cognitive role-taking, and internalized positive or negative affect over the consequences for others of one's behavior (e.g., feeling good because of positive outcomes for another when one assists or feeling guilty because not assisting would result in sustained negative conditions for another; Eisenberg-Berg 1979a).

The assertion that the aforementioned categories of reasoning reflect other-oriented concern is supported by additional research in which investigators have examined the relations between moral reasoning and behavior. Among younger children, the only other-oriented category used with any frequency is concern with others' physical, psychological, or material needs. This type of reasoning has been positively related to preschoolers' and elementary-school children's prosocial behaviors (particularly costly acts of assistance), whereas hedonistic reasoning has been negatively related (Eisenberg, Boehnke, Schuhler, and Silbereisen 1985; Eisenberg, Pasternack, Cameron, and Tryon 1984; Eisenberg and Shell 1986; Eisenberg, Shell, Pasternack, Lennon, Mathy, and Beller 1987; Eisenberg-Berg and Hand 1979; Larrieu and Mussen 1986). Moreover, higher level moral reasoning (including other-oriented reasoning of various sorts as well as other types of reasoning) has been associated with adolescents' helping behaviors (Eisenberg-Berg 1979b).

In a number of studies Eisenberg and her colleagues have also examined gender differences in prosocial moral reasoning. One of these studies is a longitudinal study in which children have been followed from 4 to 5 years of age to 11 to 12 years (Eisenberg, Lennon, and Roth 1983; Eisenberg-Berg and Roth 1980; Eisenberg, et al., 1987); other studies were cross-sectional (Eisenberg and Shell 1986; Eisenberg-Berg 1979a; Eisenberg-Berg and Neal 1981) or involved only one age group (Eisenberg et al. 1984; Eisenberg-Berg and Hand 1979). Using these data, it is possible to determine whether or not there are gender differences in prosocial moral reasoning, especially in the use of other-oriented types of reasoning, and the age at which any such gender differences emerge.

Consistent with the notion that any gender differences in prosocial moral reasoning would develop over time as a consequence of differential socialization, we have found little evidence of gender differences in prosocial moral reasoning prior to age 11. The only exception is for pragmatic reasoning; boys verbalize more of such reasoning in elementary school than do girls (Eisenberg et al. 1987), although not prior to age 7 to 8 (Eisenberg et al. 1983). However, gender differences in reasoning become more evident in the late elementary-school years and in adolescence.

Specifically, we have data in two studies that are consistent with the view that girls are more other-oriented in their prosocial moral reasoning than are boys. The first study is the aforementioned longitudinal study; in this research, gender differences in sympathetic and role-taking reasoning became apparent by the late elementary school years. These two types of reasoning were not used with any frequency until 9 to 10 years of age and use of both types of reasoning increased from 7 to 8 years of age to 11 to 12 years of age for girls, but not boys. Moreover, girls used significantly more role-taking reasoning than did boys.

In a cross-sectional study involving children in grades 2, 4, 6, 9, 11, and 12, Eisenberg (1977; Eisenberg-Berg, 1979a) found little evidence of a gender difference in overall level of reasoning. However, males and females differed somewhat in the particular categories of reasoning they used. Among the elementary schoolchildren, boys verbalized more pragmatic and direct reciprocity concerns than did girls, but only when discussing reasons for not assisting another. There were no gender differences in reasoning about decisions to assist. For the high school students, there were more significant gender differences. When discussing reasons for assisting a needy other, males were more concerned than females with direct reciprocity and the helper's affective tie to the needy other. In contrast, females used several other-oriented, empathic categories more than did boys (concern with others' psychological needs, reference and concern with humanness, sympathetic orientation) as well as the developmentally mature category "internalized positive affect related to self-respect and living up to one's own values." There were relatively few instances in which the adolescents discussed reasons for not assisting a needy other; however, when they did, males expressed more hedonistic concerns than females.

In summary, it appears that girls are more likely than boys to express other-oriented, sympathetic, and role-taking justifications in their prosocial moral judgment. However, this difference does not seem to emerge until approximately 11 to 12 years of age. Whether or not this difference becomes stronger and is maintained throughtout adulthood are issues for future research.

CONCLUSIONS

In our research on vicarious, other-oriented emotional responses (e.g., empathy, sympathy) and prosocial moral judgment, we have obtained some evidence consistent with the view that females are more oriented toward others' needs and emotions than are males. However, the differences we have obtained (with the exception of those for questionnaire indexes of sympathy, empathy, and personal distress) generally have not been large, and account for a relatively small amount of the variance in individuals' emotional responding and moral reasoning. Thus, there appears to be a need not only to determine the origins of the gender differences in prosocial moral reasoning and vicarious emotional responding (biological and socialization), but also to examine factors that account for individual differences in these types of responses within males and within females. Only then will we have a deeper understanding of the roots of caring and an other-orientation.

REFERENCES

Allen, J. G., and Haccoun, D. M. (1976). Sex differences in emotionality: A multi-dimensional approach. *Human Relations* 29: 711–720.

Barnett, M. A., Howard, J. A., King, L. M., and Dino, G. A. (1980). Antecedents of empathy: Retrospective accounts of early socialization. *Personality and Social Psychology Bulletin* 6: 361–365.

Baumrind, D. (1986). Sex differences in moral reasoning: Response to Walker's (1984) conclusion that there are none. *Child Development* 57: 511–521.

Birnbaum, D. W., and Chelmelski, B. E. (1984). Preschoolers' inferences about gender and emotion: The mediation of emotionality stereotypes. *Sex Roles* 10: 505–511.

Birnbaum, D. W., Nosanchuk, T. A., and Croll, W. L. (1980). Children's stereotypes about sex differences in emotionality. *Sex Roles* 6: 435–443.

Block, J. H. (1973). Conceptions of sex role: Some cross-cultural and longitudinal perspectives. *American Psychologist* 28: 512–526.

———. (1976). Assessing sex differences: Issues, problems, and pitfalls. *Merill-Palmer Quarterly* 22: 283–308.

Brabeck, M. (1983). Moral judgment: Theory and research on differences between males and females. *Developmental Review* 3:274–291.

Brody, L. R. (1985). Gender differences in emotional development: A review of theories and research. *Journal of Personality* 53: 102–149.

Bryden, M. P. (1979). Evidence of sex-related differences in cerebral organization. In *Sex-related differences in cognitive functioning.* (pp. 121–143), ed. M. A. Wittig and A. C. Petersen. New York: Academic Press.

Buck, R. (1983). Emotional development and emotional education. In *Emotion: Theory, research, and experience*, Vol. 2 (pp. 259–292), eds. R. Plutchik and H. Kellerman. New York: Academic Press.

Chodorow, N. (1978). *The reproduction of mothering.* Berkeley: University of California Press.

Colby, A., and Damon, W. (1983). Listening to a different voice: A review of Gilligan's *In a different Voice. Merrill-Palmer Quarterly* 29: 473–481.

Colby, A., and Kohlberg, L., eds. (1987). *The measurement of moral judgement.* Vol. 1. New York: Cambridge Press.

Condry, J., and Condry, S. (1976). Sex differences: A study of the eye of the beholder. *Child Development* 47: 812–819.

Dunn, J., Bretherton, I., and Munn, P. (1987). Conversations about states between mothers and their young children. *Developmental Psychology* 23: 132–139.

Eisenberg, N. (1977). The development of prosocial moral judgment and its correlates. *Dissertation Abstracts International* 37: 4,753B. (University Microfilms No. 77-444.)

Eisenberg, N., Boehnke, K., Schuhler, P., and Silbereisen, R. K. (1985). The development of prosocial behavior and cognitions in German children. *Journal of Cross-Cultural Psychology* 16: 69–82.

Eisenberg, N., Fabes, R. A., Bustamante, D., Mathy, R. M., Miller, P. A., and Lindholm, R. (1988). Differentiation of vicariously induced emotional reactions in children. *Developmental Psychology* 24: 237–246.

Eisenberg, N., and Lennon, R. (1983). Sex differences in empathy and related capacities. *Psychological Bulletin* 94: 100–131.

Eisenberg, N., Lennon, R., and Roth, K. (1983). Prosocial development in childhood: A longitudinal study. *Developmental Psychology* 19: 846–855.

Eisenberg, N., McCreath, H., and Ahn, R. (1988). Vicarious emotional responsiveness and prosocial behavior: Their interrelations in young children. *Personality and Social Psychology Bulletin* 14: 298–311.

Eisenberg, N., and Mussen, P. (1978). Empathy and moral development in adolescence. *Developmental Psychology* 14: 185–186.

Eisenberg, N., Pasternack, J. F., Cameron, E., and Tryon, K. (1984). The relations of quantity and mode of prosocial behavior to moral cognitions and social style. *Child Development* 55: 1479–1485.

Eisenberg, N., Schaller, M., Fabes, R. A., Bustamante, D., Mathy, R. M., Shell, R., and Rhodes, K. (In press). The differentiation of personal distress and sympathy in children and adults. *Developmental Psychology.*

Eisenberg, N., and Shell, R. (1986). Prosocial moral judgment and behavior in children: The mediating role of cost. *Personality and Social Psychology Bulletin* 12: 426–433.

Eisenberg, N., Shell, R., Pasternack, J. F., Lennon, R., Beller, R., and Mathy, R. M. (1987). Prosocial development in middle childhood: A longitudinal study. *Developmental Psychology* 23: 712–718.

Eisenberg-Berg, N. (1979a). Development of children's prosocial moral judgment. *Developmental Psychology* 15: 128–137.

————. (1979b). The relationship of prosocial moral reasoning to altruism, political liberalism, and intelligence. *Developmental Psychology* 15: 87–89.

Eisenberg-Berg, N., and Hand, M. (1979). The relationship of preschoolers' reasoning about prosocial moral conflicts to prosocial behavior. *Child Development* 50: 356–363.

Eisenberg-Berg, N., and Neal, C. (1981). The effects of person of the protagonist and costs of helping on children's moral judgment. *Personality and Social Psychology Bulletin* 7: 17–23.

Eisenberg-Berg, N., and Roth, K. (1980). The development of children's prosocial moral judgment: A longitudinal follow-up. *Developmental Psychology* 16: 375–376.

Fabes, R. A., Eisenberg, N., Miller, P., and Fultz, J. (1988). Mothers' attitudes towards emotional expressiveness and children's emotional responsiveness. Paper presented at the annual meeting of the National Council on Family Relations, November, Philadelphia, PA.

Fagot, B. I. (1981). Stereotypes versus behavioral judgments of sex differences in young children. *Sex Roles* 7: 1,093–1,096.

Feshbach, N. D. (1975). The relationship of child-rearing factors to children's aggression, empathy, and related positive and negative social behaviors. In *Determinants and origins of aggressive behavior*, eds. J. DeWit and W. W. Hartup. The Hague, Netherlands: Mouton.

———. (1982). Sex differences in empathy and social behavior in children. In *The development of prosocial behavior* (pp. 315–358), ed. N. Eisenberg. New York: Academic Press.

Freud, S. (1925/1950). Some psychical consequences of the anatomical distinction between the sexes. In *Sigmund Freud: collected papers*, Vol. 5 (pp. 186–197), ed. and trans. J. Strachey. London: Hogarth.

Gibbs, J. C., Arnold, K. D., and Burkhart, J. E. (1984). Sex differences in the expression of moral judgment. *Child Development* 55: 1,040–1,043.

Gilligan, C. (1977). In a different voice: Women's conceptions of self and of morality. *Harvard Educational Review* 47, 481–517.

———. (1982). *In a different voice: Psychological theory and women's development*. Cambridge, MA.: Harvard University Press.

Gilligan, C., and Attanucci, J. (1988). Two moral orientations: Gender differences and similarities. *Merrill Palmer Quarterly* 34: 223–237.

Grief, E. (1984). Developmental antecedents of sensitivity to emotions. Progress report to NIMH.

Grief, E., Alvarez, M., and Ulman, K. (1981) Recognizing emotions in other people: Sex differences in socialization. Paper presented at the Biennial meeting of the Society for Research in Child Development, April, Boston, MA.

Hall, J. A. (1978). Gender effects in decoding nonverbal cues. *Psychological Bulletin* 85: 845–857.

Hoffman, M. L. (1977). Sex differences in empathy and related behaviors. *Psychological Bulletin* 34: 712–722.

Huston, A. (1983). Sex typing. In *Handbook of child psychology*, Vol. 4 (pp. 387–468), ed. P. Mussen. New York: John Wiley and Sons.

Izard, C. (1977). *Human emotions*. New York: Plenum Press.

Kemper, T. D. (1978). *A social interactional theory of emotions*. New York: John Wiley and Sons.

Kohlberg, L. (1976). Moral stage and moralization: the cognitive-developmental approach. In *Moral development and behavior: Theory research, and social issues* (pp. 84–107), ed. T. Lickona. New York: Holt, Rinehart and Winston.

Larrieu, J., and Mussen, P. (1986). Some personality and motivational correlates of children's prosocial behavior. *Journal of Genetic Psychology* 147: 529–542.

Lazarus, R. S. (1982). Thoughts on the relations between emotions and cognitions. *American Psychologist* 37: 1,019–1,024.

Lennon, R., and Eisenberg, N. (1987). Gender and age differences in empathy and sympathy. In *Empathy and its development* (pp. 195–217), eds. N. Eisenberg and J. Strayer. Cambridge: Cambridge University Press.

Lennon, R., Eisenberg, N., and Carroll, J. (1983). The assessment of empathy in early childhood. *Journal of Applied Developmental Psychology* 4: 295–302.

Lewis, M., and Michalson, L. (1983). *Children's emotions and moods*. New York: Plenum Press.

Lyons, N. P. (1983). Two perspectives: On self, relationships, and morality. *Harvard Educational Review* 53: 125–145.

Maccoby, E., and Jacklin, C. (1974). *The psychology of sex differences*. Stanford: Stanford University Press.

Malatesta, C. Z., and Haviland, J. M. (1982). Learning display rules: The socialization of emotion in infancy. *Child Development* 53: 991–1,003.

Moss, H. A. (1974). Early sex differences and mother-infant interaction. In *Sex differences in behavior* (pp. 149–164), eds. R. C. Riedman, R. M. Riehart, and R. L. Vande Wiele. New York: John Wiley and Sons.

Parsons, T., and Bales, R. F. (1955). *Family, socialization, and interaction processes*. New York: Academic Press.

Plutchik, R. (1980). A general psychoevolutionary theory of emotion. In *Emotion: Theory, research, and experience* Vol. 1 (pp. 2–22) eds. R. Plutchik and H. Kellerman. New York: Academic Press.

Reinisch, J. M., and Karow, W. G. (1977). Prenatal exposure to synthetic progestins and estrogens: Effects on human development. *Archives of Sexual Behavior* 6: 257–288.

Rest, J. R. (1979). *Development in judging moral issues*. Minneapolis, MN.: University of Minnesota Press.

Shields, S. A. (1987). Women, men, and the dilemma of emotions. In *Sex and gender* (pp. 229–250), eds. P. Shaver and C. Hendreck. Newbury Park, CA.: Sage.

Shennum, W. A., and Bugental, D. B. (1982). Development of control over affective expression and nonverbal behavior. In *Development of nonverbal behavior in children*, ed. R. S. Feldman. New York: Springer and Werlog.

Walker, L. J. (1984). Sex differences in the development of moral reasoning: A critical review. *Child Development* 55: 677–691.

———. (1987). *Moral orientations: A comparison of two models*. Paper presented at the biennial meeting of the Society for Research in Child Development, April, Baltimore.

Wiesenfeld, A. R., Whitman, P. B., and Malatesta, C. Z. (1984). Positive sensitivity to infants: Evidence and support of an empathy concept. *Journal of Personality and Social Psychology* 46: 118–124.

8

Ethical Sensitivity and Moral Reasoning among Men and Women in the Professions

Muriel J. Bebeau and Mary Brabeck

The view that males and females differ in essential traits has been used to argue that men and women should be assigned to different societal roles (Lewin 1984; Rosenberg 1982). Historically, the perceptions that women lack the masculine traits of instrumentality, assertiveness, logical reasoning, detachment, and autonomy have been viewed as barriers to a woman's success in male-dominated fields (e.g. medicine, law, dentistry, higher level management) (Kaufman 1984). Historically, characteristics such as caring, sensitivity to others' needs, empathy, and concern about relationships have been viewed as "feminine" virtues by philosophers and "feminine" traits by psychologists. It has been argued that these characteristics especially equip women for the maternal role (Cancian 1987; Shields 1975; 1984) and certain professional roles (e.g., nursing and teaching, roles that involve nurturing and care) (Ehrenreich and English 1978).

Recently, however, some writers (e.g., Friedman 1988; Levine 1970) have suggested that feminine traits are especially valuable in male-dominated professions such as medicine and dentistry. The belief that women would enhance these professions through their relationship-oriented qualities (Levine 1970) suggests that women ought to be encouraged to enter male-dominated professions. This view is buttressed by Gilligan (1982) and other feminist theorists (Chodorow 1978; Lyons 1983; this volume; Martin 1985; this volume; Miller 1976; Noddings 1984; this volume). These writers do not challenge the belief that males and females differ in virtues and morality. Rather, they argue that theories of moral reasoning, and related test instruments, should put more value on "feminine" qualities and concerns. Reminiscent of Jane Addam's (1902) claim at the turn of the century that social progress depended on the unique moral insights of women, Gilligan (1982, 1986) has argued that an adequate moral theory is revealed by attending to "a different [feminine] voice."

There is evidence of the ubiquity of these stereotypes regarding masculine and feminine virtues and abilities (Bem 1974; Broverman et al., 1972; Chafetz 1978). Such gender differences, if they in fact exist, would have important implications for the education of people in the professions, as both relationship-oriented qualities and impartial, principled reasoning abilities are important for professionalism. However, recent suggestions (Gilligan 1982) that women score lower on tests of moral reasoning such as Kohlberg's, which emphasizes abstract reasoning and appeals to principles of justice at higher levels, is problematic because moral reasoning has been shown to be an important correlate of clinical performance (Sheehan et al. 1980).

What is the evidence to support the existence of gender differences? How can such differences be characterized? What evidence is there that moral theories and related test instruments are biased because they fail to attend to the different voice Gilligan identifies as an ethic of care? In this chapter we will review the literature that examines these questions. We will describe a recent four-component theoretical model of moral development (Rest 1983) that led us to investigate gender differences in an aspect of morality that is separate from moral reasoning. Specifically, we examined gender differences in situation-embedded ethical sensitivity among students aspiring to the dental profession. We will describe the instrument used to measure ethical sensitivity among dental students, the Dental Ethical Sensitivity Scale (Bebeau and Rest 1982) and present the results of our empirical work. Finally, we will argue that our empirical results suggest a reinterpretation of Gilligan's gender-related theory, an explanation for the conflicting results in other studies of male and female differences in moral development, and productive new directions for educators and for future research on the ethic of care.

REVIEW OF LITERATURE

People do believe that males and females differ in morality. Girls and women have a reputation among teachers, peers, and parents for being more helpful and empathic (Block 1984; Hoffman 1977; Shigetomi, Hartmann, and Gelfand 1981) and females report themselves to be more empathic and altruistic than males (Eisenberg and Lennon 1983; Eisenberg, Fabes, and Shea, this volume). Moreover, males expect females to make moral decisions from a more emotional perspective while seeing male morality as based on law and order reasoning (Bussey and Maughan 1982) and both male and female students classify care morality as "feminine" and justice morality as "masculine" (Ford and Lowery 1986). While self perceptions are not necessarily associated with overt behavior, the stereotype suggesting "a splitting of love and work that relegates expressive capacities to women while placing instrumental abilities in the masculine domain" (Gilligan 1982, p. 17) persists.

These views regarding male and female differences were carried into expectations of females entering the professions. In the early 1970s it was argued that the entrance of women into male-dominated professions would enhance the professions, principally because women would bring "feminine" qualities that would make the professions more person-oriented (Levine 1970). However, studies of successful academic psychologists (Helmreich et al. 1980) and of aspiring dentists (Bebeau and Loupe 1984) suggest that men and women with the qualifications to enter the professions are very similar to each other in perceptions of instrumentality and expressiveness, and do not describe themselves in the stereotypic ways observed in the general population. Women who aspire to the professions describe themselves as more instrumental than women in the general population, and men describe themselves as more expressive than do men in the general population (Bebeau and Loupe 1984).

Gilligan suggests that the expressive capacities of women influence the ways women reason about moral issues. She criticizes Kohlberg's (1969) theory because, she says, at the highest levels of his model the moral concern of females, the ethic of care, is omitted. She argues that women who have a greater concern with maintaining relationships are more likely to be scored at stage 3, the stage of mutual interpersonal expectations, relationships and conformity; males' concern with issues of justice would lead them to score at stage 4, the social system and conscience maintenance stage. Further, Gilligan asserts that hypothetical dilemmas assess logic and abstract reasoning which are more characteristic of male reasoning. Females, she argues, are excluded from the highest stages of the model because their reasoning is more particularistic and contextual.

There is evidence that logic, analytic ability and abstract reasoning are perceived as masculine traits (Broverman et al. 1972; Chafetz 1978; Lloyd 1983). However, evidence from observations of behavior does not support the stereotype (cf., Maccoby and Jacklin 1974; Linn and Petersen, 1985; Sherman 1978). If Gilligan's claim that females' contextual reasoning results in deflated scores on moral reasoning tests that assess abstract thought, we would find women scoring lower than males on the two measures of moral reasoning most commonly used, the Moral Judgment Interview (MJI) (Colby, Kohlberg, Gibbs, and Lieberman 1983) and the Defining Issues test (DIT) (Rest 1979).

To date, the literature examining gender differences in moral reasoning as defined by Kohlberg's theory do not support Gilligan's claim. Walker (1984; 1986; Walker and deVries 1985; Walker, deVries, and Trevethan 1987) has conducted a series of studies using meta-analysis to determine the effect of gender on MJI scores. He has consistently reported small effect sizes. In a recent report of a meta-analysis of 80 studies with a total of 152 samples, involving 10,637 subjects given the MJI, Walker (1986) reported that males did not score significantly higher than females. The Cohen's *d* to assess the mean effect size revealed that gender accounted for one twentieth of 1 percent of the variance in moral reasoning ($r^2 = .0005$). Baumrind (1986), a critic of Walker's work, also reported that when the effects of education are controlled, findings of gender differences in MJI scores are eliminated.

Meta-analysis (Thoma 1986) of 56 samples of over 6,000 male and female subjects who responded to the DIT yielded similar results. Thoma reported that at every age and educational level, females scored significantly higher than males, but less than half of 1 percent of the variance in DIT scores could be attributed to gender. Further, he found that education was 500 times more powerful in predicting moral judgment level than gender. These results have been supported by narrative reviews (Brabeck 1983) and by longitudinal studies that have reported that females are as likely as males to advance in the sequential order of development predicted from Kohlberg's theory (Snarey, Reimer, and Kohlberg 1985; Walker, 1989).

These results indicate that females use concepts of justice in making moral judgments as often as their male counterparts. Females are as likely as males to resolve moral issues in which individuals have competing claims, by appealing to abstract principles of justice. However, it has been argued that these studies do not necessarily undermine Gilligan's claim that Kohlberg's theory of moral reasoning is biased, because of flaws in the scoring schemes and design of the stimulus materials. With respect to the scoring scheme, Smetana (1984) argued that the Kohlbergian scoring schemes, in particular the MJI, do not include an ethic of care at all stages, thus one could not expect to find gender differences. The assumption made here is that care and justice are two distinct and separate moralities. In contrast, Kohlberg (Kohlberg, Levine, and Hewer 1983) has claimed that care is included in justice reasoning. A careful review of the MJI scoring criteria, that have been in use since 1978 (Colby et al. 1983) show that levels of relationship, caring, and interpersonal trust are considered norms and elements that are applied at each stage of the MJI scoring scheme. With respect to bias in stimulus materials, Walker (1989) showed that the ethic of care has been reliably identified and scored in studies using the dilemmas from the Kohlberg measure. It remains for future investigators to assess Kohlberg's claim that care and justice are indivisible (see also, Higgins, this volume). Nevertheless, researchers have attempted to design new measures and modify existing measures to examine care and justice as separate orientations as described by Gilligan. Studies examining claims about gender differences in the care/justice moral orientations must be interpreted cautiously since these studies are few, often employ small samples, and use different measures of moral orientation. However, there is a body of literature available that suggests the following conclusions.

First, the ethic of care can be identified in people's responses. The ethic of care has been identified and reliably scored in response to both real-life dilemmas (i.e., when subjects identify a personally experienced dilemma and discuss it) and hypothetical dilemmas (i.e., when subjects discuss a hypothetical story dilemma, such as whether or not Heinz should steal a drug to save his wife's life) (Langdale 1986; Lyons 1983; Pratt, Golding, and Hunter 1984; Rothbart, Hanley, and Albert 1986; Walker et al. 1987; Walker 1989). This suggests that the ethic of care identified by Gilligan is an identifiable aspect of people's moral responses.

Second, most studies indicate the majority of people, both males and females, use both the care and justice orientation (Gilligan and Attanucci 1988; Rothbart, Hanley, and Albert 1986; Walker et al. 1987). Thus, both males and females have been found to be concerned about the potential pain others might suffer, and to consider human relationships important moral considerations.

Third, studies examining the hypothesis that moral orientation is gender related yield inconsistent findings. Some studies that posed hypothetical moral dilemmas report no significant differences between males' and females' moral orientations (Rothbart, Hanley, and Albert 1986; Walker et al. 1987); other studies report females more likely to use a care orientation and males to use a justice orientation (Langdale 1986). Two studies that scored care-response and justice-rights responses on versions of the DIT that were modified to include care issues (Friedman, Robinson, and Friedman 1987; Pratt and Royer 1982), failed to support Gilligan's claims that males are more concerned with individual rights and women with care and concern for relationships. Furthermore, Ford and Lowery (1986) found no gender differences in students' ratings of the extent to which they used the response (care) and rights (justice) orientations. Interpretation of these studies is made difficult by the diverse ways in which care and justice orientations are measured. It must also be noted that it has not yet been empirically demonstrated that the "rights-justice" orientation measured in these studies are valid measures of Kohlberg's construct of justice moral reasoning.

Fourth, use of moral orientation appears to be related to the type of moral dilemmas being resolved. This conclusion is drawn from reviewing the studies that have used the Lyons' (1983) standardized scoring scheme to examine moral orientation by asking subjects to identify a personally experienced moral dilemma and to describe how they resolved it (Gilligan and Attanucci 1988; Lyons 1983; Langdale 1986; Rothbart et al. 1986; Walker et al. 1987). While there is inconsistency among these studies (e.g., Walker et al. 1987, did not find gender differences in moral orientation), and while most males and females used both orientations, females showed a preference for the care orientation and males for justice in self-identified moral dilemmas.

However, some researchers (Higgins, Power, and Kohlberg 1984; Nunner-Winkler 1984; Rothbart et al. 1986) report that the choice of orientation is related not to the gender of the respondent but to the type of dilemma discussed. For example, Higgins et al. (1984) report that a dilemma concerning helping another student is likely to elicit a care orientation; a dilemma about a theft is associated with justice considerations. Furthermore, Walker et al. (1987) report that while there were no gender differences in the types of "real life" moral dilemmas children identified, women reported more "personal" moral dilemmas and men more "impersonal" dilemmas. Women were more likely to raise family-related issues than men; men were more likely to raise work-related issues. These results may be due to differences in what males and females focus on as critical in defining a situation as a moral issue. The focus of moral concerns may be influenced by the activities and roles that are central in a person's life at any given time (e.g., Ruddick 1984).

Our literature review revealed that there is little difference in the ways males and females reason about the moral ideal; both principles of justice and principles of care are invoked in deciding what one ought to do to resolve a hypothetical moral dilemma. However, the differences we found in studies of self-defined moral conflicts suggest that males and females may be focusing on different issues. In a related study, Brabeck and Weisgerber (1988) asked male and female college students to describe their responses to the same real-life event, the explosion of the Challenger spacecraft. They found that while males and females did not differ in level or type of affective response, they focused on different aspects of the event. Women reported spontaneously focusing on more of the person-centered aspects of the tragedy while men reported the technological aspects were more salient. However, Brabeck and Weisgerber did not measure moral reasoning. Ford and Lowery (1986) suggest that to examine whether or not females focus on issues of relationship, responsibility, and care in defining a conflict as moral, "it seems necessary to return to a standardized . . . format." In order to examine whether males and females differ in their focus on care or justice in defining a conflict as moral, we used a standardized test (described later) to examine gender differences in situation-embedded ethical sensitivity. Rest's (1983) recently described theory of the components of morality offered a theoretical model for testing our hypothesis.

A NEW PERSPECTIVE ON MORAL DEVELOPMENT: ETHICAL SENSITIVITY

Rather than arguing that the Rawlsian concept of justice as fairness exemplified by Kohlberg's stage theory excludes concern for care, connectedness, and harmony, one might search for the presence or absence of care, as it relates to other components of morality. Rest (1983) has described ethical sensitivity as the first of a four component model of morality. Ethical sensitivity (Component 1) is the identification of the salient ethical aspects of a dilemma. The processes of Component 1 are used prior to (Component

2) formulating a morally defensible course of action, for example, appealing to principles of justice. These processes are followed by Component 3, distinguishing between moral and nonmoral values and committing to the moral value, and Component 4, executing and implementing a plan of action that resolves the moral problem effectively.

According to Rest, ethical sensitivity (Component 1) can be distinguished from principled moral reasoning (Component 2). While the latter involves "determining what course of action would best fulfill a moral ideal, what *ought* to be done in the situation" (Rest 1983, p. 561) the former involves interpreting the situation and identifying "possible courses of action in a situation that affect the welfare of someone else" (p. 559). Moral sensitivity includes making inferences from individuals' verbal and nonverbal behaviors, identifying what others want or need, anticipating their reactions to one's attempt to help, and responding with appropriate affect.

NEW MEASURE OF MORAL SENSITIVITY: DESCRIPTION AND SUMMARY OF STUDIES OF VALIDITY AND RELIABILITY

Bebeau and Rest (1982) have developed a measure of ethical sensitivity (Rest's Component 1) to assess the ability of dentists to identify and interpret typical ethical problems that arise in dental practice. Four dramas, based on a study of the recurrent ethical problems in the practice of dentistry (Bebeau, Reifel, and Speidel 1981) are presented in the Dental Ethical Sensitivity Test (DEST).

Synopsis of DEST Dramas

The Judy Radiwich Case. Dr. Oldham is about to retire. He plans to sell his practice to Dr. Young, a recent graduate. Dr. Oldham observes Dr. Young as he considers a treatment for Judy Radiwich, a young woman from a prominent family in the community. They have been patients of Dr. Oldham's practice for years. As they discuss the treatment, a difference of opinion develops on what treatment should be recommended. Dr. Oldham insists that Dr. Young follow his advice.

The Jim Lohman Case. Jim Lohman has a toothache that requires endodontic treatment. He needs much other work, but has little money. Several options are presented, but he has difficulty making a decision.

The Margaret Herrington Case. Ms. Herrington has recently moved to a new city. Her new dentist notices advanced periodontal disease and traumatic occlusion on the crown of a molar, and moderate periodontal disease around five other crowns. Upon inquiry, the dentist is informed that the crowns were placed about two years ago. Margaret appears to be unaware of the periodontal disease. The dentist believes the crowns cannot be salvaged; they must be replaced. Margaret does not have dental insurance.

The Sandy Johnson Case. Sandy Johnson is a young woman with serious dental and oral health problems. She is extremely thin. She is interested in improving her appearance as she believes she is getting a new job. She resists any discussion of nutrition and describes her annoyance with her mother who is, as she describes it, constantly nagging her about eating.

The dramatizations consist of dialogues between a dentist and client, such as might occur in a dental office. These tape-recorded dramas serve as stimulus materials that subjects hear. Subjects are tested on what they identify as the problems presented. This is accomplished by having subjects enter into a dialogue with a drama character. The subject's dialogue and subsequent responses to interview questions, which ask about the assumptions and perspectives underlying the student's responses, are tape recorded.

The interviews are transcribed and scored for the degree of sensitivity to several characteristics of the patient and sensitivity to the responsibilities of the dentist. The four interviews are scored by assigning ratings from one to three to indicate the degree of recognition of each of 34 criteria (seven to ten criteria per drama). Summing across the four dramas yields a minimum score of 34 and a maximum of 102 points.

It is noteworthy that the scoring criteria were developed in collaboration with practicing dentists and moral philosophers. We believe that both issues of fairness (justice) and concerns for harmony, connectedness, and nonviolence (care) are reflected in the criteria. In fact, it was the practicing dentists who most clearly articulated the ethic of care. Examples include: concerns for giving information about the status of health in a way that will cause the least hurt; concerns that giving bad news about standard care could so undermine trust in the profession that the individual may stop seeking care, and thus be doubly harmed; and, an overriding concern for resolving problems in a way that maintains relationships between dentists and patients, and between patients and the profession.

DEST Reliability

The reliability of the DEST is reported in several studies, most recently summarized in Rest, Bebeau, and Volker (1986). Item agreement averaged 86.5 percent in one study, and 89.9 percent in another. Agreement between raters, that is, correlations calculated for drama subscores, averaged .87 for the four dramas. Test-retest correlations over several weeks averaged .68 at the individual drama level, and by the Spearman-Brown formula is estimated at .90 for the test as a whole.

The Validity of Moral Sensitivity as a Theoretical Construct

Research exploring the properties of measures of moral sensitivity in professional situations is still underway. However, findings from Volker's (1984) study of moral sensitivity, using a measure designed for counseling psychologists, and studies of dental students' moral sensitivity using the DEST (see Rest et al. 1986), indicate the following:

1. The content validity of both measures is well established, and the scoring criteria are sufficiently well defined to produce adequate interrater reliability.

2. Moral sensitivity correlates only moderately with DIT scores (in the .2 to .5 range), which indicates that Component 1 processes are separate from Component 2 processes. Thus, morality is not a single, unitary process. It is possible for a person to be skilled at interpreting the ethical issues in a situation (Component 1), but unskilled at working out a balanced view of a moral solution (Component 2), and vice versa.

3. There is evidence for both convergent and divergent validity. Both Bebeau and Volker asked experienced clinicians to rate transcripts of subject responses on moral sensitivity without knowledge of their respective scoring schemes. These ratings were compared to scores produced by the scoring system. Volker reported a correlation of .95, indicating agreement between his formalized measure of moral sensitivity and the more intuitive judgments of experienced clinicians, thus demonstrating convergent validity. He also offered evidence of divergent validity in that moral sensitivity scores were negatively ($-.52$) correlated with verbosity. DEST scores correlated .69 with the practitioner's intuitive rankings of moral sensitivity and only correlated in the .20 to .40 range with measures of verbal fluency, technical knowledge, and word count of subjects' responses.

4. Data collected from a sample of counseling psychologists and from several samples of dental students indicate that individuals vary greatly in moral sensitivity. Further, moral sensitivity, as measured by the DEST, has been shown to improve with deliberate instruction (Zimney 1986).

5. Although each DEST drama contributes specific variability in moral sensitivity, evidence of the degree of internal consistency of the measures is high enough (Cronbach alphas ranging from .70 to .78) to enable us to study moral sensitivity as a construct.

EMPIRICAL INVESTIGATION OF MORAL REASONING AND ETHICAL SENSITIVITY

Our examination of Rest's Component 2, the moral reasoning (DIT scores) and Component 1, moral sensitivity (DEST score) among male and female dental students draw upon data from a number of on-going studies of professional ethical development. We expected that women dental students would be more sensitive to the potential hurt experienced by the dental patient, more concerned about the affective state of the patient, and more aware of the interpersonal issues. Thus, we predicted that females would identify more ethical aspects of dilemmas that professionals face when treating dental patients than would males. Research has shown that differential socialization (e.g., Block 1984) has led women to place greater emphasis on interpersonal relationships. Females have also been found to be more accurate than males in decoding nonverbal cues about another person's affective state (Eisenberg and Lennon 1983; Eisenberg et al., this volume) and more likely to appeal to empathic role taking to justify stage 3 moral reasoning (Gibbs, Arnold, and Burkhart 1984). Thus, we hypothesized that while males and females would not differ in their reasoning after a moral dilemma had been defined (Component 2), they would differ in sensitivity to ethical issues (Component 1). Research described earlier, which found that differences in moral orientation were related to the type of situation subjects identified as moral dilemmas, supports our prediction.

The advantage of studying gender differences in this professional school context using the DEST are as follows: 1) extensive data on background variables are available, so the equivalency of the male and female groups can be established, and 2) the DEST is a well-validated measure that, though not specifically designed to test Gilligan's conceptions of different moral orientations, makes extensive use of these concepts in assessing an ability which is thought to be an essential component of moral behavior. The DEST scoring scheme provides an overall indication of sensitivity and specific items assess recognition of issues of care and issues of justice. Both relationship and justice issues are contained in all the DEST dramas, but two dramas present situations in which there is a high degree of tension between care and justice. Analysis of specific items in these dramas seemed particularly appropriate for determining gender preferences for these issues.

Analysis of data from several data sets enabled us to 1) compare male and female dental students' moral reasoning; 2) examine gender differences in ethical sensitivity, particularly the ability to identify ethical problems which are embedded in situations frequently encountered by dentists; 3) analyze whether male dental students are more likely to recognize justice issues and female students more likely to identify care issues as salient; 4) examine differences between males and females in the priority assigned care and justice issues; and 5) determine whether students can integrate both care and justice issues in their responses to ethical problems after training.

To determine whether women would attend to care issues more than men, we selected a subset of the existing DEST scoring criteria where issues of care and justice seemed to be in tension (see DEST Scoring Manual [Bebeau and Rest 1982], items 11.C. and 11.D. of the Radiwich Case, and items I.E. and I.F. of the Herrington Case). The Radiwich and Herrington dramas (described earlier) presented clues to a conflict between relationship and justice in a way that expert clinicians find difficult to resolve (Bebeau, Reifel, and Speidel 1981). By applying existing criteria, it is possible to assess the degree to which students attended to each issue. For example: In the Judy Radiwich drama, technical clues about Judy Radiwich's dentition, combined with Judy's expressed concern for aesthetics ought to alert the student to recommend a treatment alternative that is contrary to the wishes of Dr. Oldham. A tension develops between the young dentist's duty to give priority to the patient's rights (the fairness issue) and his wish to maintain harmony with Dr. Oldham, a colleague, elderly man, and a person from whom he hopes to purchase the practice (the care issue). In the Margaret Herrington drama, clues are presented that ought to alert the listener to the fairness issue: Margaret should not have to pay again for work that does not meet professional standards and appears to have caused harm to her periodontal health. Likewise, the dialog ought to alert the listener to the care issue: because Margaret's previous dentist helped her overcome her apprehension (she liked and trusted him), and because she cares deeply about her oral health, news about her health status and the previous inferior dental work is likely to be upsetting and may interfere with her confidence in both the old and new dentist and could influence her decision to continue with dental care.

The selected items from the Radiwich and Herrington dramas were scored for the degree to which students recognized each issue. The scoring manual includes discrete descriptions for a three-point scale, where 3 = clear recognition and 1 = no recognition. Judges are permitted to use a 1.5 and 2.5 category for responses that fall short of the next criterion. Then, responses were examined to see whether men and women students had a tendency to prioritize care over justice or vice versa. Responses to each drama were classified into one of the following categories: Clearly recognized both issues (e.g., scores a 2.5 or 3 on care, and 2.5 or 3 on justice); Shows some, but equal, recognition of both issues; Prioritizes justice over care; Recognizes justice/ignores care (e.g., scores a 3 on justice, a 1 on care); Prioritizes care over justice; Recognizes care/ignores justice; Ignores both issues. See Moen (1987) for exact coding rules.

University of Minnesota dental students complete the DIT and the DEST as part of course requirements for the curriculum in professional ethics. The DIT was first administered in 1979, and data are currently available for all entering freshmen and several advanced level groups. DEST scores were first obtained in 1981 and protocols have been collected for 145 beginning and over 500 advanced level students. Typically, protocols are scored by a cadre of practicing dentists who use the Scoring Manual (Bebeau and Rest 1982), and provide individual feedback to students.

In addition to DEST and DIT scores, data are available on undergraduate GPA, scores on the Dental Aptitude Test, dental school GPA, clinical performance ratings, and other demographic variables. Clinical performance ratings, assigned by clinic directors and codirectors at the end of the senior year, were selected for gender comparison because the scale includes assessment of interpersonal skills, personal characteristics, and professional abilities that are relevant to Gilligan's theoretical claims. The 20 item six-point Likert scale used at Minnesota is similar to scales used in medical schools, but Minnesota faculty achieve remarkably high interrater reliability when compared with other studies of the reliability of such measures (Meetz, Bebeau, and Thoma 1988). Further, clinical performance ratings of Minnesota students predict timely completion of dental school requirements, a criterion faculty believe is an important predictor of success in practice. Clinical ratings are not related to preadmissions criteria nor to dental school GPA.

We conducted a number of analyses to investigate gender differences in ethical sensitivity (Component 1), measured by the DEST and moral reasoning (Component 2), measured by the DIT. (These results and additional discussion can be found in Bebeau and Brabeck 1987). A summary of the results follows.

A meta-analysis of seven groups of male and female dental students (first year and third year) who took the DIT prior to implementing an ethics curriculum, indicated effect sizes (Cohen's d) that varied from $-.45$ to $.53$ across the samples. Collapsing across the seven samples indicated a mean of 47.20, $SD = 12.64$ for 593 males, and a mean of 47.60, $SD = 12.97$ for 184 females, with an effect size of $d = .03$. This difference is lower than the average effect size ($d = .21$) reported by Thoma (1986), suggesting that men and women dental students are very similar in moral reasoning ability.

Since educational factors have been shown to account for differences in moral judgment (Thoma 1986), we needed to determine the equivalency of the 196 male and 44 female students before analyzing gender differences in ethical sensitivity. No significant differences were observed on undergraduate GPA (Males $M = 3.21$, $SD = .36$; Females $M = 3.23$, $SD = .35$); Dental Aptitude Scores (Males $M = 4.85$, $SD = 1.47$; Females $M = 4.50$, $SD = 1.36$); or, Clinical Performance Ratings (Males $M = 90.14$, $SD = 15.33$; Females $M = 89.81$, $SD = 14.57$). On the two clinical performance subscales, where we thought gender differences might appear, that is, personal attributes and interpersonal abilities, women achieved slightly higher scores (mean differences of .5 and 1.00 point respectively), but the differences were not significant.

Our meta-analysis replicates previous reports (Thoma 1986) that gender differences in the ability to resolve hypothetical dilemmas, using principles of justice as measured by the DIT, are small. Females and males do not differ in their ability to reason abstractly about moral issues (Component 2).

Next, we examined gender differences in ethical sensitivity (Component 1). Transcripts of 196 men and 44 women (class of 1985 and 1986) who took the DEST in the spring of their junior year were analyzed by two raters, both dentists, who established their interrater reliability following the procedures described in Bebeau, Rest, and Yamoor (1985). Agreement ranged from 78 percent to 91 percent, with an average of 86 percent across the 34 items. Interrater reliability, calculated for the total score for each drama, ranged from .78 to .91, with an average reliability of .83. The mean DEST score for 44 women in the two classes was significantly higher $p < .002$ than for the 196 men. An estimate of the effect size (Cohen's d) indicates a moderate effect, $d = .51$ overall, and analysis of differences at the drama level indicates that each drama is contributing to the overall effect. Item analysis indicates that women scored significantly higher than men on only four of the 34 items, equal to or somewhat higher than men on 23 items, somewhat lower than men on six items, and significantly lower on one item. Thus, the observed gender differences resulted from a cumulative effect that was not attributable to any identifiable cluster of items.

One possible explanation for the greater ethical sensitivity of women might be attributed to prior experience or training within the profession. Equivalency of males and females on clinical performance and attitudes, academic achievement, and previous professional experience was established prior to testing for gender differences in DEST scores. However, Coombs (1976) reported that prior experience in dentistry was a determining factor in career choice for 58 percent of the women entering dental school in the early 1970s. Therefore, a comparison of DEST scores of the 20 women who had such prior experience or training with those who did not was made; it was not significant, $p < .67$.

Women dental students showed significantly greater sensitivity to the ethical issues contained in professional dilemmas than did their male colleagues. These differences cannot be attributed to differences in clinical performance, academic achievement or prior experience in the profession, or to prior training or experience in the related professions, dental hygiene, nursing or dental assisting. Thus, there appears to be a gender difference in what Rest has identified as Component 1, the ability to identify the ethical issues of a dilemma.

To further investigate gender differences in ethical sensitivity, we compared mean recognition scores by gender for the care and justice items and examined how the men and women prioritized the care and justice issues in each of the two cases from the DEST. Complete transcripts were available for 87 women who completed the DEST as juniors between 1981 and 1985. An equal number of men from each class was randomly selected for the gender comparison. Analyses of recognition of care and justice issues in the two DEST dramas were conducted by a dental student who practiced rating items and comparing ratings with the test developer until 80 percent agreement was consistently achieved. Samples selected to test interrater reliabilities achieved 90 percent agreement. Comparison of mean recognition scores by gender for care and justice items indicated one significant finding. The women achieved significantly higher scores ($M = 2.26$, $S.D. = .77$) than the men ($M = 2.02$, $S.D. = .85$) on recognition of the justice issue in the Radiwich case. Cohen's d estimate of the effect size, indicated a small to moderate effect (.36) favoring women. A chi-square revealed that women did not prioritize care over justice issues more frequently than men, nor did men prioritize justice over care issues more frequently than women. In fact, trends were not even in the expected direction, as 36 percent of the men compared with 29 percent of the women recognized care but ignored the justice issue (see Table 8.1). Based on the item analysis described earlier and the prioritization of care and justice concerns differences in ethical sensitivity appear to

Table 8.1
Prioritization of Care and Justice Issues by Gender for Two Dramas

Number of Responses Per Category

Prioritization Categories	Men (N=87)			Women (N=87)		
	Judy Radiwich	Margaret Herrington	Cases Combined	Judy Radiwich	Margaret Herrington	Cases Combined
Complete Integration	16	2	18 (10%)	10	4	14 (8%)
Some Integration	16	10	26 (15%)	14	6	20 (11%)
Care over Justice	4	3	7 (4%)	4	1	5 (3%)
Care Ignore Justice	13	38	51 (29%)	25	38	62 (36%)
Justice over Care	23	6	29 (17%)	20	9	29 (17%)
Justice Ignore Care	9	3	12 (7%)	9	5	14 (8%)
Ignores both Issues	6	25	31 (18%)	5	24	29 (17%)

result from greater sensitivity to a wide range of patient characteristics and professional responsibilities rather than to a greater propensity on the part of women to attend to issues of care.

Consistent with the literature we reviewed on gender differences in moral reasoning (Component 2), women who were at the same educational level as their male counterparts did not give greater priority to issues of care, nor were there differences in the ability of males and females to integrate care and justice issues. A concern to educators is the fact that only about one-fourth of the students give equal recognition to both issues and 17.5 percent of the students failed to recognize either issue. Since this integration is necessary for adequate identification of the moral aspects of a professional dilemma, these results suggest a need for training and led us to examine significant changes in ethical sensitivity following completion of a professional ethics course.

Forty juniors (38 males and 2 females) who completed the DEST before and after a five week course in Professional Problem Solving were selected from Zimney's (1986) sample and categorized according to preference for care and justice issues in the Herrington and Radiwich cases. We examined changes in subjects' integration of care and justice issues following instruction. The chi-square ($df = 6$) was 19.31, $p < .001$, ($N = 40$) and significant changes occurred in two categories: 1) the proportion of students who integrated care and justice after instruction was significantly greater, and 2) the number of students who no longer ignored both care and justice issues was greatly reduced (see Table 8.2). Zimney's (1986) study showing significant change in DEST scores following instruction indicates that moral sensitivity is an ability that can be developed. Our results confirm that higher levels of integration of care and justice can be achieved following instruction.

The DEST was designed to measure ethical sensitivity in a dental context, but we believe it could be used to explore gender differences with other populations. Technical knowledge of dentistry is prerequisite to a full understanding of the complexity of the ethical issues, but the measure has been used successfully to assess sensitivity of entering freshmen (Bebeau, Rest, and Yamoor 1985), who presumably lacked technical knowledge. Alternatively, the methodology employed in the DEST could be used to develop profession-specific tests to study ethical sensitivity among males and females in other professions.

This line of research also suggests that much may be gained by understanding morality as multi-faceted. The findings of researchers that women are socialized to be more empathic, altruistic, and nurturing (Block 1984; Eisenberg et al., this issue) may be useful in examining the source of the gender difference we observed. Other fruitful areas of study may be to explore gender differences in commitment to moral values (Component 3), or the ability to effectively execute moral intentions (Component 4 in Rest's

Table 8.2
Percent of Students (*N* = 40) Integrating Care and Justice Issues Before and After Instruction

Number of Responses Per Category

Prioritization Categories	Before Instruction			After Instruction		
	Judy Radiwich	Margaret Herrington	Cases Combined	Judy Radiwich	Margaret Herrington	Cases Combined
Complete Integration	1	6	7 (9%)	2	11	13 (16%)
Some Integration	0	1	1 (1%)	2	5	7 (9%)
Care over Justice	1	2	3 (4%)	0	1	1 (1%)
Care Ignore Justice	4	20	24 (30%)	3	14	17 (21%)
Justice over Care	8	3	11 (14%)	10	5	15 (19%)
Justice Ignore Care	13	0	13 (16%)	20	1	21 (26%)
Ignores both Issues	13	8	21 (26%)	3	3	6 (8%)
Total			80 (100%)			80 (100%)

[1983] system). Clearly, those engaged in the education and development of professionals need to examine how students are being trained to attend to the care and justice issues in moral dilemmas they will confront within their profession.

REFERENCES

Addams, J. (1902). *Democracy and social ethics*. New York: Macmillan and Co.

Baumrind, D. (1986). Sex differences in moral reasoning: Response to Walker's (1984) conclusion that there are none. *Child Development* 57: 511–21.

Bebeau, M. J., and Brabeck, M. M. (1987). Integrating care and justice issues in professional moral education: A gender perspective. *Journal of Moral Education* 16: 189–203.

Bebeau, M. J., and Loupe, M. (1984). Masculine and feminine personality attributes of dental students and their attitudes toward women's roles in society. *Journal of Dental Education* 48: 309–14.

Bebeau, M. J., and Rest, J. R. (1982). *The dental ethical sensitivity test*. Center for the Study of Ethical Development, Burton Hall, University of Minnesota.

Bebeau, M. J., Rest J. R., and Yamoor, C. M. (1985). Measuring dental students ethical sensitivity. *Journal of Dental Education* 49: 225–35.

Bebeau, M. J., Reifel, N. M., and Speidel, T. M. (1981). Measuring the type and frequency of professional dilemmas in dentistry. *Journal of Dental Research* 60 (Abstract #891) 532.

Bem, S. L. (1974). The measurement of psychological androgyny. *Journal of Consulting and Clinical Psychology* 43: 155–162.

Block, J. H. (1984). *Sex role identity and ego development*. San Francisco: Jossey-Bass.

Brabeck, M. (1983). Moral judgment. Theory and research on differences between males and females. *Developmental Review* 3: 274–91.

Brabeck, M., and Weisgerber, K. (1988). Responses to the Challenger tragedy: Subtle and significant gender differences. *Sex Roles* 19: 639–50.

Broverman, I. K., Vogel, S. R., Broverman, D. M., Clarkson, F. E., and Rosenkrantz, P. S. (1972). Sex-role stereotypes: A current appraisal. *Journal of Social Issues* 28: 59–78.

Bussey, K., and Maughan, B. (1982). Gender differences in moral reasoning. *Journal of Personality and Social Psychology* 42: 701–6.

Cancian, F. (1987). *Love in America: Gender and self-development*. Cambridge, MA: Cambridge University Press.

Chafetz, J. S. (1978). *Masculine feminine or human*. Itasca, IL: F. E. Peacock Publishers.

Chodorow, N. (1978). *The reproduction of mothering: Psychoanalysis and the sociology of gender*. Berkeley, CA: University of California Press.

Colby, A., Kohlberg, L., Gibbs, J., and Lieberman, M. (1983). A longitudinal study of moral judgment. *Monographs of the Society of Research in Child Development* 48: (1–2, Serial No. 200).

Coombs, J. A. (1976). Factors associated with career choice among women dental students. *Journal of Dental Education* 40: 724–32.

Ehrenreich, B., and English, D. (1978). *For her own good: 150 years of the experts' advice to women*. Garden City, NY: Anchor Press/Doubleday.

Eisenberg, N., and Lennon, R. (1983). Sex differences in empathy and related capacities. *Psychological Bulletin* 94: 100–31.

Ford, M. R. and Lowery, C. R. (1986). Gender differences in moral reasoning: A comparison of the use of justice and care orientations. *Journal of Personality and Social Psychology* 50: 777–83.

Friedman, E. (1988). Changing the ranks of medicine:Women MDs. *Medical World News*, April 25, pp. 57–68.

Friedman, W. J., Robinson, A. B., and Friedman, B. L. (1987). Sex differences in moral judgments? A test of Gilligan's theory. *Psychology of Women Quarterly* 11: 37–46.

Gibbs, J. C., Arnold, K. D., and Burkhart, J. E. (1984). Sex differences in expression of moral judgment. *Child Development* 55:1,040–43.

Gilligan, C. (1982). *In a different voice: Psychological theory and women's development*. Cambridge, MA: Harvard University Press.

———. (1986). Reply by Carol Gilligan. *Signs: Journal of Women in Culture and Society* 11: 324–33.

Gilligan, C. and Attanucci, J. (1988). Two moral orientations: Gender differences and similarities. *Merrill-Palmer Quarterly* 34: 223–37.

Helmreich, R. C., Spence, J. T., Beane, W. E., Lucker, G. W., and Matthews, K. A. (1980). Making it in academic psychology: Demographic and personality correlates of attainment. *Journal of Personality and Social Psychology* 39: 869–908.

Higgins, A., Power, C., and Kohlberg, L. (1984). The relationship of moral atmosphere to judgments of responsibility. In *Morality, moral behavior and moral development*, eds W. M. Kurtines and J. L. Gewirtz. New York: John Wiley and Sons.

Hoffman, M. L. (1977). Sex differences in empathy and related behavior. *Psychological Bulletin* 84: 712–22.

Kaufman, D. R. (1984). Professional women: How real are the recent gains? In *Women: A feminist perspective*, ed. J. Freeman. Mountain View, CA: Mayfield Publishing Co.

Kohlberg, L. (1969). Stage and sequence: The cognitive-developmental approach to socialization. In *Handbook of socialization theory and research*, ed. D. A. Goslin. Chicago: Rand McNally.

Kohlberg, L., Levine, C., and Hewer, A. (1983). *Moral stages: A current formulation and a response*. Basel: Karger.

Langdale, S. (1986). A re-vision of structural-developmental theory. In *Handbook of moral development*, ed. G. L. Sapp. Birmingham, AL: Religious Education Press.

Levine, P. T. (1970). Distaff dentists. *Journal of Dental Education*, 34: 352–57.

Lewin, M. (1984). *In the shadow of the past: Psychology portrays the sexes*. New York: Columbia University Press.

Linn, M. C., and Petersen, A. C. (1985). Facts and assumptions about the nature of sex differences. In *Handbook for achieving sex equity through education*, ed. S. S. Klein. Baltimore: The Johns Hopkins University Press.

Lloyd, G. (1983). Reason, gender and morality in the history of philosophy. *Social Research* 50: 490–513.

Lyons, N. (1983). Two perspectives: On self, relationships, and morality. *Harvard Educational Review* 53: 125–45.

Maccoby, E. E., and Jacklin, C. N. (1974). *The psychology of sex differences*. Stanford, CA: Stanford University Press.

Martin, J. R. (1985). *Reclaiming a conversation*. New Haven, CT: Yale University Press.

Meetz, H.K., Bebeau, M. J., and Thoma, S. J. (1988). The validity and reliability of a clinical performance rating scale. *Journal of Dental Education* 52: 290–97.

Miller, J. B. (1976). *Toward a new psychology of women*. Boston: Beacon Press.

Moen, T. K. (1987). Gender differences in dental students' ability to recognize ethical issues. Unpublished manuscript, University of Minnesota, School of Dentistry.

Noddings, N. (1984). *Caring: A feminine approach to ethics and moral education*. Berkeley, CA: University of California Press.

Nunner-Winkler, G. (1984). Two moralities? A critical discussion of an ethic of care and responsibility versus an ethic of rights and justice. In *Morality, moral behavior and moral development*, eds. W. M. Kurtines and J. L. Gewirtz. New York: John Wiley and Sons.

Pratt, M. W., Golding, G., and Hunter, W. J. (1984). Does morality have a gender? Sex, sex role, and moral judgment relationships across the adult life span. *Merrill-Palmer Quarterly* 30: 321–40.

Pratt, M. W., and Royer, J. M. (1982). When rights and responsibilities don't mix. Sex and sex-role patterns in moral judgment orientation. *Canadian Journal of Behavioral Science* 14: 190–204.

Rest, J.R. (1979). *Development in judging moral issues*. Minneapolis: University of Minnesota Press.

———. (1983). Morality. In *Carmichael's Manual of Child Psychology, Volume 3: Cognitive Development*, ed. P. Mussen. (556–629), New York: John Wiley and Sons.

Rest, J. R., Bebeau, M. J., and Volker, J. (1986). An overview of the psychology of morality. In *Moral development: Advances in research and theory*, ed. J. R. Rest. New York: Praeger Publishers.

Rosenberg, R. (1982). *Beyond separate spheres: Intellectual origins of modern feminism*. New Haven, CT: Yale University Press.

Rothbart, M. K., Hanley, D., and Albert, M. (1986). Gender differences in moral reasoning. *Sex Roles: A Journal of Research* 15: 645–53.

Ruddick, S. (1984). Maternal thinking. In *Mothering: Essays in feminist theory*, ed. J. Trebilcot. Totowa, NJ: Rowman & Allanheld Pub.

Sheehan, T. J., Hustad, S. D., Candee, D., Cook, C. D., and Bergen, M. (1980). Moral judgment as a predictor of clinical performance. *Evaluation in the Health Professions* 3: 393–404.

Sherman, J. (1978). *Sex-related cognitive differences*. Springfield, IL: C. C. Thomas.

Shields, S. (1975). Functionalism, Darwinism, and the psychology of women: A study in social myth. *American Psychologist* 30: 739–54.

———. (1984). "To pet, coddle and do 'do for'" Caretaking and the concept of maternal instinct. In *In the Shadow of the past: Psychology portrays the sexes*, ed. M. Lewin. NY: Columbia University Press.

Shigetomi, C. C., Hartmann, D. P., and Gelfand, D. M. (1981). Sex differences in children's altruistic behavior and reputations for helpfulness. *Developmental Psychology* 17: 434–37.

Smetana, J. (1984). Morality and Gender: A Commentary on Pratt, Golding, and Hunter. *Merrill-Palmer Quarterly* 30: 341–48.

Snarey, J., Reimer, J., and Kohlberg, L. (1985). The development of socio-moral reasoning among kibbutz adolescents: A longitudinal cross-cultural study. *Developmental Psychology* 21: 3–17.

Thoma, S. (1986). Estimating gender differences in the comprehension and preference of moral issues. *Developmental Review* 6: 165–80.

Volker, J. M. (1984). Counseling experiences, moral judgment, awareness of consequences, and moral sensitivity in counseling practice. Ph.D. diss., University of Minnesota.

Walker, L. J. (1989). A longitudinal study of moral reasoning. *Child Development* 60: 157–166.

———. (1986). Sex differences in the development of moral reasoning: A rejoinder to Baumrind. *Child Development* 57: 522–26.

———. (1984). Sex differences in the development of moral reasoning: A critical review. *Child Development* 55: 677–91.

Walker, L. J., and deVries, B. (1985). Moral stages/moral orientations: Do the sexes really differ? In C. Blake (Chair), Gender difference research in moral development, Symposium conducted at the meeting of the American Psychological Association, Los Angeles.

Walker, L. J., deVries, B., and Trevethan, S. D. (1987). Moral stages and moral orientations in real life and hypothetical dilemmas. *Child Development* 58 (3): 842–58.

Zimney, L. (1986). Unpublished Data. University of Minnesota.

9

The Caring Self:
Social Experiences of Power
and Powerlessness

M. Brinton Lykes

> The very theme of difference, whatever the differences are represented
> to be, is useful to the oppressing group . . . any alleged feature
> attributed to an oppressed group is used to imprison this group within
> the boundaries of a Nature which, since the group is oppressed, ideolog-
> ical confusion labels 'nature of oppressed person' . . . to demand the
> right to Difference without analyzing its social character is to give back
> the enemy an effective weapon.
>
> Minha-ha 1987, p. 18

Among the many issues that Carol Gilligan's (1982) work *In a Different
Voice* raised for feminist theorists and psychologists was the possibility that
women speak in a "different moral voice," that is, that women respond to
an "imperative to care" and that this response has been absent from and
devalued by ethical, and, more specifically, psychological theories of moral
development. Irrespective of the scholarly assessment of the validity or
generalizability of her findings (see this volume for a number of critiques
and extensions of her work), the popular response to her book suggests, at
least, that Gilligan was speaking to a set of issues that touched deeply many
middle- and upper-middle class educated U.S. women. Resonating to the
experiences and dilemmas confronting the women she interviewed, many
women saw their own conflicts between meeting their own needs and caring
for others. Through the description of the "different voice" Gilligan
provided important "validation" for these women.

Gilligan developed a framework for describing women's different voice
in her three-level typology of care. (See Puka, this volume for an
elaboration of the levels.) Throughout her work, and more particularly in
the work of several of her colleagues (see, for example, Lyons 1983, and this
volume), she assumes that differences in moral reasoning are related to

differences in self-understanding. More specifically, attachment, relationship, and interdependence form a contextual web through which a woman comes to understand herself and to define moral behavior.

Of the several questions left unanswered by her exploratory research, and by Gilligan's subsequent work, is a discussion of the sources of the differences between women and men that she posits. She suggests in her introduction that she makes "No claims . . . about the origins of the differences described or their distribution in a wider population, across cultures, or through time. Clearly, these differences arise in a social context where factors of social status and power combine with reproductive biology to share the experiences of males and females and the relations between the sexes" (Gilligan 1982, p. 2). Indeed her empirical evidence does not permit a broader claim. Yet her decision not to address the social character of these differences yields precisely the kind of problem suggested by Minha-ha (1987) above. More specifically, to demand that we acknowledge and affirm this difference without analyzing its social character is, at the very least, to leave Gilligan and her followers vulnerable to a biological interpretation of the sources of the gender difference in moral decision-making, that is, that girls/women are "naturally" more caring than boys/men. This reasoning slips quickly from description to prescription and women become, as suggested in an earlier analysis by Jean Baker Miller (1976), constrained to traditional forms of caring or service. While confronting ethicists, feminists, and psychologists once again with the conundrum of difference, Gilligan's work challenges us to examine the "ethic of care" more critically and to seek further clarification of the "different voice" that she hypothesizes. Without such work the theory runs the risk of reinforcing rather than liberating many of the existing norms concerning women's and men's moral behavior (see Puka and Houston, this volume, for more extensive discussions of this point).

This chapter takes up Gilligan's unanswered question about the sources of differences in ethical reasoning. More specifically, it summarizes earlier work on alternative theories about the self and argues that an analysis of the social character of the ethic of care through the lives of non-middle class non-white women offers an alternative understanding of women's moral thinking and action and suggests that we must seek alternative language to that of care to adequately describe women's moral thinking and behavior.

AN EMPIRICAL INVESTIGATION OF WOMEN'S SENSE OF SELF

In my own research I have explored the social character of women's sense of self, a sense that Gilligan argues focuses on social relations and the importance of interconnection. Drawing on social theorists who emphasize the centrality of a self-in-relation, (see, for example Miller 1976, 1984; Jordan 1984; Kaplan and Surrey 1984) Gilligan affirms this alternative description of the self that more adequately describes the lived experiences of the women participants in the research and clinical work of many feminist psychologists.

These theories suggest an important alternative to the dominant model of the self embedded in an assumption of autonomous individualism and to dominant psychological models of the self that emphasize autonomy, separation, and independence and ignore the inherently social character of the self. Yet they retain certain problematic characteristics that prevent the full articulation of a notion of a social self. Chodorow's (1978) argument that women are more relational and empathetic suggests that these gender differences are due to the fact that women, universally, are largely responsible for early child-care ("women's mothering is one of the few universal and enduring elements of the sexual division of labor," p. 3) and is key to accounting for gender differences in women's sense of self and in moral reasoning. Although Chodorow's argument underlies much subsequent work about both women's sense of self and women's moral reasoning, in neither body of work is it explicitly analyzed. More specifically, the dyadic relationship, particularly the mother-child relationship that is posited as core to the child's first internal representation of self and is key to the development of the child's self-understanding, is described independently of the social totality in which it is grounded.

Evidence from an empirical investigation of selected experiences of white, working, and pink collar and professional adult women and men (see Lykes 1985; Stewart and Lykes 1985) supported my argument that there are multiple notions of the self (the two which were the focus of my efforts are autonomous individualism and social individuality). It suggested that the culturally dominant notion of the self, rooted in assumptions of autonomy and independence and separation, is but one orientation to the self. A contrasting notion, social individuality, reflects a dialectical understanding of individuality and sociality grounded in an experience of social relations characterized by inequalities of power.

Notions of the self (see Lykes 1985) are embedded in and reconstructed from social arrangements. The notion of the self as an ensemble of social relations reflects the inextricable unity of individuality and sociality evidenced in a truly social sense of self. However, the most pervasive view of the self in the dominant U.S. culture, sustained by powerful, ideological, and structural forces remains that of autonomous individualism (see, e.g., Hogan 1975; Hsu 1983; Kanfer 1979; Lewis 1979; Smith 1978; Wikse 1977). Various responses to such arrangements, including among others, some form of conformity and some form of resistance, vary by social group membership and by social experiences. I did, therefore, anticipate differences in people's notions of the self deriving from social experiences both at the group level (e.g., as a member of a social group excluded from power) and at the individual level (e.g., experiences in collective activities for social change).

Multiple indexes were used to measure social individuality at various levels of cognitive functioning. Four indexes—cognitive-perceptual styles, apperception, ideology, and reasoning about moral dilemmas—were selected as apertures on the self as social individuality.

As expected the four measures were intercorrelated, supporting the hypothesis that the notion of the self, social individuality, is reflected at these four levels. The analyses also supported my hypothesis that selected life-experiences, some that vary due to membership in a social grouping (e.g., gender or occupational level) and others rooted in early or current life activities (e.g., participation in collective activities), are systematically associated with one's conceptualization of the self. Interviews with women in this sample suggested additional differences in the ways in which women whose notion of the self resembles that of social individuality and those whose notion of self resembles that of autonomous individualism. For example, the former group, whom I refer to as social individuals, are more likely than the autonomous individuals to evidence both a widening circle of relationship from childhood to adulthood, (including family, friends, neighborhood, and community) and a tendency to participate actively in these communities, in addition to work and family responsibilities. Social individuals tend to describe themselves in terms of relatedness to friends, family, neighborhood, and society. Their frequent acknowledgment of political and social differences with family or friends suggests that interconnection does not negate particularity or difference.

The interview material confirmed findings in the quantitative analyses and supports the expectations that women are more likely to perceive the interrelation of self and others and the self-defining/defined nature of social experiences than men. This is particularly true among women working at the lower ends of the occupational ladder and/or those who have in some way resisted institutional forces that exclude them from power. Involvement in activities that focus on the transformation of oppressive structures, in which one acts on a belief in the interdependence of all people or through which one is reinforced in one's sense of belonging through community, may serve both to concretize an abstract sense of oneself as an "ensemble of social relations" and to provide a place where consciousness and action converge.

Although exploratory, my research (Lykes 1985) suggests several important directions for future research and theorizing about gender in psychological research on the self. The effort to identify a theory of the self rooted in an analysis of the *essential* qualities of the mother-child relationship overlooks the complex set of relationships that constrain that experience and that define its meaning for social participants. Identification of female mothering as a nearly universal experience and as the critical and foundational relationship for understanding one's sense of self is problematic. This is not to suggest that knowing and understanding the mother-child attachment/separateness is not critical for understanding the self and our notions of the self. Nor do I mean to argue against a position that suggests that all women may share some characteristics, even biologically based characteristics (Lewis 1976), in common. Rather I am arguing that a failure to focus on the particularity of mother-child relating and the cross-cultural and cross-contextual variations in the meaning of adult-child attachment-separateness reduces the highly variable social bases for our notions of the self to a base of individualism. This can only support an individualistic understanding of the self. Such efforts are also embedded in inherently flawed efforts to reduce biology or individuality and environment or sociality to separate elements (Lowe and Hubbard 1983).

Analyses of the relationship of the social organization of material life and the mother-child experience provide evidence of the importance of collective experiences for developing a notion of the social self. Leacock's (1983) descriptions of societies organized communally in kin groups where networks of exchange relations are egalitarian in form, children are cared for by the kin-based collective and women are not economically dependent on men, suggest a link between the social organization of material life and the parent-child experience (see also Turnbull's, 1984 description of the Mbuti for a similar point). If, as Chodorow argues, the sex/gender system (see also Rubin 1975) is a sociocultural construction, surely mothering in kin-based collectives and in hierarchically ordered nuclear families was and is differentially experienced and enacted. Knowledge of such differences is critical to an understanding of the individual's developing sense of self grounded in an analysis of the mother-child relationship.

Carol Stack (1974) makes a similar point in her descriptions of the ties of kinship and friendship in a poor, black urban community in the United States in the twentieth century. The sense of self that emerges from these kin-based networks where the "recognized mother, the 'mama' . . . determines the child's kinship affiliations through females" (p. 49) is not of a single autonomous individual interacting but of a coacting network of relationships embedded in an intricate system of social exchanges and obligations. Stack argues that these experiences of mother and child reflect this people's creative response to the harsh economic realities of poverty and racism.

Joseph (Joseph and Lewis 1981) refers to black mothers' and daughters' experiences as a "dynamic dyad," as a "communication/interaction process" (p. 82). The black daughters in her national survey describe their mothers in terms of qualities understood within a context of community, for example, "her creativity and talents in keeping the family together in spite of the difficulties she has to face" (p. 125). Although white daughters in a comparison sample frequently mentioned the same characteristics, that is "creativity" or "talent," their descriptions reflected a tendency to abstract their mothers from a context, an attempt to capture some essential quality or trait possessed by an individual. For the black women in Joseph's sample, mothering and daughtering are particular, dynamic changing processes whose meaning develops within a broader social and historical context. The framework developed by white psychologists to describe the mother-daughter relationship fails to capture adequately this quality which is reflective of both the strong traditions of black family patterns rooted in African cultures and the structional oppression of racism that both constrains the resources available to blacks for parenting and shapes the messages they communicate early on to their children. (see, Joseph 1984, for a similar point, Bell-Scott and Guy Sheftall 1984, for a fuller treatment of black mothers and daughters.)

Further, despite the important description of a woman's sense of self as intrinsically relational, that is, as codetermined by a mutually affirming relationship that confirms " . . . the validity of your own self as a person-in-relationship" (Kaplan 1984, p. 10), the basis upon which this understanding rests remains individual, interpersonal experiences (see Lykes 1985 for a further development of this point). Such interactionist views of the self-in-relation support a lopsided focus on attachment, while the self can only be fully understood with equal focus on separateness. Concepts describing the self developed in a socially grounded personality theory would focus on the articulation of individuality in the activity of social interrelatedness.

Community or collective experiences are thus fundamental to the articulations of individuality and relationship that emerge. The experiential basis for the idea of the self-in-relation is the community, grounded in the totality of social relations. This contrasts both with the dominant view of autonomous individualism and with the view reflected in societies whose dominant resolution of the individual-society problem in collectivism results in the dissolution or negation of individuality (see, for example, Taylor 1972, on the "group-mindedness" of the Zuni; Tuan 1982, on the "sense of group self" of the Kaingang; Dumont 1970, 1980, on India). An elaboration of experiences of "community" and "collectivity" in our society and of the ways in which these experiences are constrained by differential access to power and resources (i.e., of the material fabric of these experiences) provides a critical base for developing a notion of the self as social. Such concepts, in turn, alter our views of various human experiences as, for example, the discussion of mothering presented here suggests, or as evidenced in Fine's (1983-84) contextually based reanalysis of the experience of rape.

CARING FOR THE SELF/OTHER

A woman's decision not to report or press charges against her assailant after being raped has been described by some as a failure to cope, and, more damningly, as a failure to care for herself, to resist gender oppression and, more specifically, violence against women. Fine's (1983-84) analysis of the class, race, and gender oppression that contextualizes Altamese Thomas's decision not to accuse the man who raped her reveals the ways in which her action is an affirmation of community ties. Fine presents Altamese's critique of the criminal justice system's discrimination against blacks, particularly black males, and her own analysis of the biases woven into the "taking-control-yields-coping" formulations that dominate much psychological theory about women and violence. Altamese's understanding of who she is, of who her people are, is reflected in her "choice" and constructed by both the traditional forms of family and community (with its roots in the African experiences) and by the structures of oppression under white capitalism. It is only careful attention to the social character of the difference between Altamese's response and that reflected in dominant formulations that yields an understanding of Altamese's act and suggests the need for a corrective to the earlier formulations.

Altamese's resolution of her "moral dilemma" (whether or not to report her assailant) takes on even bolder relief in the context of Eugene's (this volume) discussion of a liberational ethic of care. Eugene's analysis is grounded in and contributes to an understanding of black women's and men's confrontation with and resistance to the structures of racism/sexism/capitalism and of the importance of African and Afro-American traditions and practices to understanding contemporary black strategies for survival. Eugene suggests that her description of black women's resistance illustrates level 3 of Gilligan's ethic of care. Drawing on the evidence she presents and the arguments developed here I suggest that Eugene's work, rather than confirming Gilligan's typology, turns it on its head. Responsiveness to the self and to others is not "connected" as Gilligan argues. To posit a connection is to imply and confirm a separation, that is, that they are separate entities and must be brought together (by the individual woman who develops this ethic of care). Eugene's analysis boldly demonstrates that for black women "the other" is not other in our classic understanding of opposition. Rather "other" and "self" are co-constituting, co-defining. There is no self out of connection, no connection without self in the resistance to structural oppression. This affirmation of community not only reframes Gilligan's ethic of care but further suggests a reframing of dominant analyses of women, particularly black women, as the other. It suggests the problematic of the very construct of self. That is, there is no self-construct independent of the social context; there is no self-understanding divorced from history and from material conditions. (This is consistent with Seigfried's [this volume] and Tronto's [1987] arguments that sensitivity to context is essential to moral deliberations.)

This seemingly abstract construction is enfleshed in Eugene's descriptions of black women's activity. Eugene's "liberational ethic of care" is grounded in the self-other dialectic and implies a dialectic between justice and care. The ethic underlying the activity she describes and characteristic of Altamese's decision-making is not in opposition to the ethic of justice. Rather it redefines what is meant by justice, what is meant by care. Neither the self-in-relation nor the ethic of care accurately describe the self-in-community and the structural oppression within and against which black women act.

Although Eugene's analysis focuses on black feminists, her description of black community is echoed by other black authors who have sought to document the community's experiences. James Langston Gwaltney's (1980) self-portrait of black America identifies certain values that define core black culture. There is a commitment to honesty, to "telling the truth," an emphasis on respect for others and for their choices, a generosity motivated by the knowledge that you might need help someday, and a belief "in the solidarity born of a transgenerational destination of [their] subordination" (p. xxvii). Wade Nobles (1976) suggests that similar "virtues" reflect a different pattern of thought, one that is connected to a different self-concept, a view of the self that stresses a "sense of cooperation," "interdependence," and "collective responsibility."

AN ISSUE OF POWER

The question of power and of relations of power, central to my understanding of the socio-historical grounding of differing notions of the self in North American psychological theories, has become more salient as I have sought to understand Latin American women's responses to state-sponsored violence within their communities. I conducted oral history interviews with Guatemalan Indian women (see, Lykes 1986, in press) who were in exile in Mexico because of a violent counterinsurgency program launched by the Guatemalan military against its people between 1979 and 1983. Through this experience I came to understand many of the contradictions these women and their children confronted. Miles away from their traditional Indian communities and needing to hide their Indian identity to avoid deportation, they sought ways to return to their homes while beginning the slow process of constructing an alternative community in exile. They sought nurturance and security for their children while simultaneously preparing them for their hoped for return to Guatemala. Their primary concern was "the children," a concern which mothers throughout the world have shared, particularly in times of war and social upheaval. But these women were not only concerned about their "own" children. They wondered about the children of Guatemala, the more than 100,000, mostly Indian children, who had lost at least one parent between 1979 and 1983, and the millions of children being raised in a climate of violence. They wondered about the future of their country.

The understanding of their experiences and the articulation of their concerns for their community, for the future of their country, are reflected in the actions of various groups of women that have gathered throughout the world during the past 15 years. These groups demand answers to the brutal violence that has ravaged numbers of countries in the so-called developing world. In Guatemala, the Mutual Support Group for Relatives of the Disappeared (GAM) was formed in mid-1984 by a group of mothers, spouses, sisters, and daughters seeking information about their disappeared relatives.[1] Nineth Montenegro de Garcia, one of the founders, recalls:

Before the group was formed, someone very prominent came up to me and said, "Look, lady, even if you do everything you possibly can, you're never going to find your husband, and that's supposing he's alive." I told him, "Wait, you'll see; we're going to do something. . . . " Together with my mother-in-law, I began to talk to people. . . . [One was the mother of an engineer.] She was very scared; Raquelita said, "Look, one little dove all by itself doesn't do anything." But finally she came and there were three of us. And that's how it began (Hernon and Malone 1986).

For several years, during a continuing period of military dictatorship and through the transition to the current "democracy,"[2] the GAM was the only group within Guatemala to protest the horrifying human rights abuses that had resulted in the disappearances of over 30,000 people (one-third of all the disappearances of Latin America), the deaths of over 100,000 people, and the displacement of over 1 million in a country of only 8 million people (see Carmack 1988; Lykes 1988, in press; Manz 1988).

The GAM has held regular demonstrations and marches in front of the National Palace and continues to ask the government to intervene immediately to find their loved ones. They have not been allowed to protest peacefully. In April 1985 a GAM member, Rosario Godoy de Cuevas, her two-year old son, and her brother were found dead; their bodies revealed they had been tortured. This was the second attack on the GAM whose director of press relations had been tortured and killed the previous month. However, the murders of Gomez and Godoy did not intimidate the GAM members who marched less than 10 days later with approximately 1,000 supporters through downtown Guatemala City in tribute to their slain leaders.

The GAM shares similar goals to the Mothers and Grandmothers of the Plaza de Mayo in Argentina, the Association of Families of the Detained-Disappeared in Chile, and many other groups throughout the world. These organizations are made up almost entirely of women and have emerged in each of their countries at moments of intense and often continuing political repression to become the social conscience of the country. They have requested, then demanded, that the government "intervene immediately to find our loved ones" (Guatemala), that their loved ones be "brought back alive" (Argentina), or that the government "for life or for peace, tell us where they are" (Chile). Immediate responses of governments to these groups' public outcries against the disappearances and demands for truth and justice were to deny that anyone had disappeared and to call the women "Las Locas" (mad women). Yet these women have persisted in the face of official denials and other more violent repression, such as that described above.

These women have taken their private pain, the loss of a child, of a spouse, of a sibling and brought it into the public domain. It is not, as they themselves have said repeatedly, that they were not afraid. They were terribly afraid, and like many others in their country they had maintained silence about what had happened, searching quietly through existing government channels. But at some point, first in twos and threes, then in hundreds and now in thousands they gathered together to break the silence enshrouding the violation of human rights within their respective countries.

Power and State-sponsored Violence: A Refocusing of the Question

The suggestion that structured relations of power and powerlessness are central to understanding people's notions of the self and their ethical behaviors has taken on new dimensions. From an analysis of gender and economic stratification within a stable, democratic, developed country women's moral action in Latin America forces consideration of the consequences for self-understanding when confronted with massive violence that is not only tolerated by the state but, in the cases described here, directly sponsored by the state. The ideological rationale for these "cultures of death" has been the Doctrine of National Security under which governments claim to be waging a war against international communism, which is expressed domestically through local subversion, thus threatening "the nation" both externally and internally. (Subversion in these contexts is equated with the desire to secure title to one's land or feeding the poor of an inner city barrio.)

Fear immobilized much of the population during the most extreme periods of this blood bath. Women responded to these extreme forms of violence in Argentina (between 1976 and 1983), in Chile (since 1973), and in Guatemala (most recently, since the late 1970s). Women "unbalanced the silent anti-dictatorship status quo by stepping out of the family, leaving the allegedly protected environments of their homes to invade the streets with their presence . . . " (Bunster 1988, p. 485; see also, Agosin 1987; Simpson and Bennet 1985). Women have used their traditional roles as mothers strategically to protest repressive practices within military dictatorship, thereby both drawing on traditional, stereotypical definitions of femaleness and reconstructing the meaning of motherhood.

Particular strategies, such as the Chilean *arpilleras* (small wall hangings on burlap backing with superimposed figures depicting Chilean life, designed to denounce political conditions in the country), reflect even more directly how women's traditional tasks, that is, for example, stitchery, have been reconstructed as instruments of female power. The *arpilleristas* (those who design and make the *arpilleras*) have not directly challenged the traditional Chilean view of the woman as the "mainstay, the major social force governing the home, the major socializing force" (Agosin 1987, p. 32) whose power is respected in that sphere but who are not easily permitted to move from that traditional sphere. Rather they have used the conditions of their motherhood as their prime political weapon (Agosin 1987).

They have also drawn on less traditionally female strategies to assist them in their struggle for justice and for truth. The Grandmothers of the Plaza de Mayo in Argentina, seeking to look for, identify, and restitute to their life stories and to their families of origin the more than 400 Argentine children kidnapped or born in captivity to kidnapped mothers,[3] rely on the most sophisticated legal and scientific techniques to support their work (Abuelas de Plaza de Mayo 1987, 1988; Arditti and Lykes, in press). They approached the American Academy for the Advancement of Science (AAAS, Washington, DC) seeking a genetic test to confirm grandpaternity. At the urgings of the Grandmothers and with the technical contribution of the AAAS the Argentine government has established a Genetic Bank wherein the blood types of all relatives of disappeared are being recorded (Arditti 1988; Beckwith 1987; Human genetics 1984). This evidence is being used to support the Grandmother's efforts at restituting identified children to their life stories and to their families and will be available to any Argentine child who seeks to recover her/his true story. As importantly, the Grandmothers have been in the leadership of including a provision in the revision of the Declaration of the Rights of Children currently being drafted by the United Nations to guarantee any child's right to his/her identity (Child rights treaty 1988).

A full analysis of the significance of these activities within the traditional Latin American society where the social construction of femininity and machismo remain strong is beyond the scope of this chapter. Further, scholarship about women in Latin America (see, for example, Agosin 1987; Bunster 1988; Carlson 1988) documents women's traditionally conservatizing role in the political and social spheres. Within this context the mothers and grandmothers described here contrast sharply with women's dominant role of maintaining the political status quo or supporting conservative governments. (Women's role in the overthrow of Allende in Chile, for example, reflects this attitude.) Equally important is the analysis of the various contradictory roles that women have and continue to play in Latin America's dictatorships. Bunster's (1988) graphic descriptions of the network of pro-Pinochet women who currently represent "'a living affirmation,' a tacit approval of the oppressive junta regime" (p. 490) echoes Koonz's (1987) important analysis of women and the family in Nazi politics. As Bunster (1988) suggests, "we are only beginning to learn about the structural vulnerability of women who ally themselves with military governments" (p. 491). Yet within these contexts the activities of the grandmothers and mothers suggest that under certain conditions and at certain historical moments women are reconstructing definitions of mothering, definitions of care.

CONCLUSIONS

The research summarized above and the examples drawn from Latin America question the necessary connection between gender per se and alternative modes of moral decision-making or alternative notions of the self. They suggest that differences in morality and in self-understanding are grounded in social experiences of power and powerlessness, some of which are due to gender. An analysis of the social character of the diversity of women's lives expands the range of behaviors that constitute "ethical action" and demonstrates the complexity of women's social location. It further suggests the urgent need to develop an analysis of the social character of women's lives if we are to accurately understand differences among women and between women and men.

The work of the Latin American "mothers" and "grandmothers" further suggests that the effort to confront the ethical dilemmas facing women and men in the face of state-sponsored terrorism or its consequences are not so distant from those that underly contemporary U.S. theory and practice of mothering (see Arditti and Lykes, in press; Fariña, 1988; Lykes and Fariña, 1989 for a fuller discussion of these points). For example, the Grandmothers' activities strike the core of family issues and reproductive rights. They are asking some basic questions that all human beings face: What is a family? What is the status of children? Is there an inalienable human right to know one's origins? What are the implications for adoption, for children born from artificial insemination, for "surrogacy"?

Latin American "mothers" and "grandmothers" are collectively asserting the right of men, women, and children to truth, to their individual stories, to their families, and to their country. This assertion is grounded in a strategy that embraces the connections among women and men and draws on these ties to develop strategies for demanding truth and justice. One's mothering is constituted by and constitutive of ties to one's children, one's community, one's people. But these ties have been violently broken by the violations of human rights described above. Mothers and grandmothers, daughters and sisters are reconstituting them. Memory and identity become the basis for human dignity and a strategy against the danger of collective amnesia taking over the minds of people. As these women start to raise the veil of powerful and violent military systems we can get glimpses of a future where people will no longer be dispossessed, women and children turned into objects. Taken as a whole the struggles of North American white and black women and of Latin American women, despite and because of considerable "differences," strongly argue for a language about caring that accurately describes the dialectic of justice and care embodied in their struggles for truth, so clearly reflected in their work. Such language, will, of necessity, reflect an analysis of the social character of each experience.

NOTES

I would like to thank the people of Guatemala, Argentina, and Chile whose struggles I have come to know and share during the past six years. I hope that this work will contribute to our mutual understanding and search for truth and justice. Thanks also to Juan Jorge Fariña and the members of the Movimiento Solidario de Salud Mental, Buenos Aires, to the members of my Feminist Research Methodology Group, to members of the Network in Communication and Scientific Documentation in Mental Health and Human Rights, and to Rhode Island College—all of whom have contributed to the work presented here. Finally, my thanks to Mary Brabeck whose feedback on earlier drafts, and more importantly, whose encouragement and support of this work and of the people of Guatemala, have been an important resource to me.

1. Disappearance of persons constitutes a new category in the implementation of the repressive methodologies of state-sponsored terrorism, as justified by the Doctrine of National Security that has dominated Latin America during the last 20 years. The person is abducted at any moment from home or from a busy street, often in the presence of others. Shoved into a vehicle with darkened windows and driven away, the person is not arrested nor is he/she kidnapped in the sense that family are asked for something in exchange for her/his release. To the contrary, the family receives no communication; the person has disappeared. Except in rare cases most disappeared persons reappear as bodies found dumped by roadsides or in common graves, bearing signs of torture. Although successive military governments have denied involvement in disappearances, witness after witness has expressed certainty to international human rights organizations that government, police, or military personnel are responsible for these incidents. Argentina is the only Latin American country to successfully convict a small number of the thousands responsible for these heinous crimes against humanity.

2. On January 14, 1986, Vinicio Cerezo Arévalo was inaugurated Guatemala's first civilian president in 16 years, its sixth since 1898. He was quoted at the time as saying that he had less than 30 percent of the power; the military had the rest. Estimates are that the repeated coup attempts during 1988 (the most significant of which were in May and in August) have eroded his power further.

Próspero Penados del Barrio, the Archbishop of Guatemala City, confirmed the continuing repression in April 1987, when he said, ''There has been a change in government but not of those who control it. The army is the same. They keep killing many people'' (Simon 1987, p. 16). Both the Interamerican Commission of Human Rights of the Organization of American States and Amnesty International issued reports in October 1988, indicating a notable increase in human rights violations in Guatemala. Amnesty International and America's Watch, reputable independent monitors of human rights worldwide, indicate that the authors of most of these abuses are members of the security forces, dressed as civilians.

3. From 1976 to 1983, during a period of successive military juntas, 30,000 Argentines disappeared during what is known as the ''Dirty War'' in Argentina. More than 400 children were either kidnapped with their parents or born in the more than 340 secret detention camps throughout the country. Many of these children had their identities changed and were given up for adoption, often to the same military who had been involved in the torture and murder of their parents. The Grandmothers

seek to restore these children and all of the children of Argentina to the truth about their families, their origins, their roots.

REFERENCES

Abuelas de Plaza de Mayo. (1987). *Abducted children in Argentina*. (September). Available from Abuelas de Plaza de Mayo, Corrientes 3284, Piso 4, Depto "H," 1193 Capital Federal, Argentina.

———. (1988). *El secuestro-apropiación de niños y su restitución*. (July). Available from Abuelas de Plaza de Mayo, Corrientes 3284, Piso 4, Depto "H," 1193 Capital Federal, Argentina.

Agosin, M. (1987). *Scraps of life: Chilean arpilleras*. Translated by C. Franzen. Trenton, NJ: The Red Sea Press.

Arditti, R. (1988). Genetics and justice: The Grandmothers of the Plaza de Mayo enroll scientists in their struggle for human rights. *Woman of Power* 11:42-44.

Arditti, R., and Lykes, M. B. (In press). "Juliana's case": The Grandmothers of Plaza de Mayo and the kidnapped children of Argentina. *Sojourner: The Women's Forum*.

Beckwith, B. (1987). Science for human rights. *Science for the People* 19(1):6-9, 32.

Bell-Scott, P., and Guy-Sheftall, B., eds. (1984). Mothers and daughters [Special issue]. *Sage: A Journal of Black Women* 1(2).

Bunster, X. (1988). Watch out for the little Nazi man that all of us have inside: The mobilization and demobilization of women in militarized Chile. *Women's Studies International Forum* 11(5):485-491.

Carlson, M. (1988). *Feminismo!: The woman's movement in Argentina from its beginnings to Eva Perón*. Chicago, IL: Academy Chicago Publishers.

Carmack, R. M., ed. (1988). *Harvest of violence: The Maya Indians and the Guatemalan crisis*. Norman and London, OK: University of Oklahoma Press.

Child rights treaty finished, but debate isn't. (1988). *New York Times*, December 11, p. 18.

Chodorow, N. (1978). *The reproduction of mothering: Psychoanalysis and the sociology of gender*. Berkeley, CA: University of California Press.

Dumont, L. (1970). The individual as an impediment to sociological comparison and Indian history. In *Religion, politics and history in India: Collected papers in Indian sociology*, ed. L. Dumont. Paris/The Hague: Mouton Publishers.

Dumont, L. (1980/1966). *Homo hierarchicus: The caste system and its implications*. Translated by M. Sainsbury, L. Dumont, and B. Gulati. Chicago, IL: University of Chicago Press.

Fariña, J. J. (1988). Ethical and epistemological questions: Experimentation on children in Argentina. Paper presented in March at Boston College, Chestnut Hill, MA.

Fine, M. (1983-84). Coping with rape: Critical perspectives on consciousness. *Imagination, Cognition, and Personality* 3(3):249-267.

Gilligan, C. (1982). *In a different voice: Psychological theory and women's development*. Cambridge, MA: Harvard University Press.

Gwaltney, J. L. (1980). *Drylongso: A self-portrait of Black America*. New York: Random House.

Hernon, D., and Malone, B. (1986). *Guatemala: A human rights tragedy.* Washington, DC: Network in Solidarity with the People of Guatemala.

Hogan, J. (1975). Theoretical egocentrism and the problem of compliance. *American Psychologist* 30(5):533-540.

Human genetics and human rights: Identifying the families of kidnapped children. (1984). *American Journal of Forensic Medicine and Pathology* 5(4):339-347.

Hsu, F. L. K. (1983). *Rugged individualism reconsidered: Essays in psychological anthropology.* Knoxville, TN: The University of Tennessee Press.

Jordan, J. V. (1984). *Empathy and self boundaries.* (Working Papers in Progress, No. 85-05). Wellesley, MA: Wellesley College, The Stone Center.

Joseph, G. (1984). Black mothers and daughters: Traditional and new populations. *Sage: A Scholarly Journal on Black Women* 1(2):17-21.

Joseph, G., and Lewis, J., eds. (1981). *Common differences: Conflicts in black and white feminist perspectives.* Garden City, NY: Anchor Press/Doubleday.

Kanfer, F. H. (1979). Personal control, social control, and altruism: Can society survive the age of individualism? *American Psychologist* 34(3):231-239.

Kaplan, A. G. (1984). *The "self-in-relation": Implications for depression in women.* (Working Papers in Progress, No. 84-03). Wellesley College, The Stone Center.

Kaplan, A., and Surrey, J. L. (1984). The relational self in women: Developmental theory and public policy. In *Women and mental health policy* (pp. 79-94), ed. L. E. Walker. Beverly Hills, CA: Sage.

Koonz, C. (1987). *Mothers in the fatherland: Women, the family and Nazi politics.* New York: St. Martin's Press.

Leacock, E. (1983). Ideologies of male dominance as divide and rule politics: An anthropologist's view. In *Woman's nature: Rationalizations of inequality* (pp. 111-121), ed. M. Lowe and R. Hubbard. New York: Pergamon Press.

Lewis, H. B. (1976). *Psychic war in men and women.* New York: New York University Press.

Lewis, M. (1979). *The culture of inequality.* New York: New American Library.

Loew, M., and Hubbard, R., eds. (1983). *Women's nature: Rationalizations of inequality.* New York: Pergamon Press.

Lykes, M. B. (1985). Gender and individualistic vs. collectivist bases for notions about the self. *Journal of Personality* 53(2):357-383.

_____ . (1986). The will to resist: Preservation of self and culture in Guatemala. Paper presented at the International Annual Meeting of the Latin American Studies Association, October, Boston, MA.

_____ . (In press). Dialogue with Guatemalan Indian women: Critical perspectives on constructing collaborative research. In *Representations: Social constructions of gender,* ed. R. Unger. Amityville, NY: Baywood Publishing Co.

_____ . (1988). Violence and psychosocial trauma in Guatemala. Paper presented at the Annual Meeting of the American Public Health Association, November, Boston, MA.

Lykes, M. B., and Fariña, J. J. (1989). *Family engineering: Epistemology, ethics and Fascist paternity.* Unpublished manuscript. Available from first author, 1892 Beacon Street, Brookline, MA 02146.

Lyons, N. P. (1983). Two perspectives: On self, relationships, and morality. *Harvard Educational Review* 52(2):125-145.

Manz, B. (1988). *Refugees of a hidden war: The aftermath of counterinsurgency in Guatemala*. NY: State University of New York.

Miller, J. B. (1976). *Toward a new psychology of women*. Boston, MA: Beacon Press.

_____. (1984). *The development of women's sense of self*. (Working Papers in Progress, No. 84-01). Wellesley, MA: Wellesley College, The Stone Center.

Minha-ha, T. T. (1987). Difference: "A special Third World issue." *Feminist Review* 25:5-22.

Nobles, W. W. (1976). Extended self: Rethinking the so-called Negro self-concept. *Journal of Black Psychology* 2(2):15-24.

Rubin, G. (1975). The traffic in women: Notes on the "political economy" of sex. In *Toward an anthropology of women*, ed. R. R. Reiter. New York: Monthly Review Press.

Simon, J-M. (1987). *Guatemala: Eternal spring, eternal tyranny*. New York: W. W. Norton & Co.

Simpson, J., and Bennet, J. (1985). *The disappeared and the Mothers of the Plaza: The story of the 11,000 Argentinians who vanished*. New York: St. Martin's Press.

Smith, M. B. (1978). Perspectives on selfhood. *American Psychologist* 33(12): 1,053-1,063.

Stack, C. B. (1974). *All our kin: Strategies for survival in a Black community*. New York: Harper and Row.

Stewart, A. J., and Lykes, M. B., eds. (1985). *Gender and personality: Current perspectives on theory and research*. Durham, NC: Duke University Press.

Taylor, G. R. (1972). *Rethink: A paraprimitive solution*. London: Secker & Warburg.

Tronto, J. C. (1987). Beyond gender difference to a theory of care. *Signs: Journal of Women in Culture and Society* 12(4):644-661.

Tuan, Yi-Fu. (1982). *Segmented worlds and self: Group life and individual consciousness*. Minneapolis, MN: University of Minnesota Press.

Turnbull, C. M. (1984). The individual, community and society: Rights and responsibilities from an anthropological perspective. *Washington & Lee Law Review* 41(1):77-132.

Wikse, C. V. (1977). *About possession: The self as private property*. University Park, PA: Pennsylvania State University Press.

Part III

EDUCATING FOR CARE

10

Transforming Moral Education

Jane Roland Martin

THE CURIOUS CASE OF *LIFELINE*

In an analytic review of six models of moral education, the *Lifeline* program developed by Peter McPhail and his associates (1975) is characterized as "more impressive in practice than in theory" (Hersh, Miller, and Fielding 1980, p. 69). Asserting that the strength of McPhail's consideration model lies in its materials, the authors advise readers to consult other models for the rigorous theoretical treatment this "relatively comprehensive approach to moral education" lacks (p. 69). Reaffirming their concern about theory in their conclusion, they say, "If the teacher can bring to the materials the theoretical insights that other models provide (e.g., Shaver's and Kohlberg's) then the *Lifeline* program can be a valuable contribution to the enterprise of moral education" (Hersh et al. 1980, p. 72).

What is this approach to moral education whose value depends on the acquisition of an adequate theoretical framework? The guiding purpose of the *Lifeline* curriculum is "to empower the student to give and receive love" (Hersh et al. 1980, p. 52). Built around the theme of learning to care, its materials focus on understanding other people's needs and situations and being sensitive to them. Whereas Lawrence Kohlberg's (1973) cognitive development model identifies increasing maturity with greater sophistication in moral reasoning and the goal of James Shaver's (Shaver and Strong 1976) rationale building model is the development of independent moral thinking, the consideration model construes maturity as creative caring. Thus, "imaginative helping" is held to be the most mature student response to the question "What would you do?" posed by cards on which drawings portray interpersonal situations.

To which models should *Lifeline*'s friends turn for theoretical help? The candidates that Hersh and colleagues (1980) propose are Shaver's and Kohlberg's models. Yet can a curriculum that focuses on love and what Carol Gilligan (1982) has called an ethic of care, obtain theoretical help from a model that gives affect "a back seat to cognition," as reviewers say Shaver's does (Hersh et al. 1980, p. 51)? Or that focuses "a great deal of attention on reasoning" without making the linkages to emotion sufficiently clear, as they say Kohlberg's does (Hersh et al. 1980, p. 158)?

I raise these questions here not to defend McPhail's consideration model against its critics. Neither the details of the *Lifeline* curriculum nor the particulars of the rationale behind it need detain us. It is the anomalous character of this approach to moral education that interests me. Of the six models of moral education that Hersh, Miller, and Fielding review, the consideration model is the only one primarily concerned with "moral sentiments" and the only one found so lacking in theoretical support that we are told to seek help elsewhere. Moreover, there is a telling discrepancy between the assessments of McPhail's model and the other five. Dwelling on *Lifeline*'s theoretical limitations and perceiving them to be a grave defect, Hersh et al. (1980) refer us to models whose neglect of moral sentiments suggests in advance the futility of such advice. Mentioning in passing the affective limitations of the other models and perceiving them to be a minor flaw, they do not think these call for help.

We need to understand why an approach to moral education that stresses caring and love exists in a kind of theoretical limbo and why a perceived failure of other models to do justice to moral sentiments is not considered a grave defect. These are not idle concerns. In *The Fate of the Earth* Jonathan Schell says, "Formerly, the future was simply given to us; now it must be achieved" (1982, p. 174). Deriving this conclusion from his appraisal of the nuclear peril, Schell understands that to achieve the future we must do more than acknowledge an obligation to save the species; we must comprehend that obligation as "a new relationship among humans"—"a form of love," he calls it, resembling "the generative love of parents." The nuclear peril, he goes on to say, "makes all of us, whether we happen to have children of our own or not, the parents of all future generations" (Schell 1982, p. 175). Schell is absolutely right that the nuclear peril requires us to rethink human relationships and, in addition, our relationship to the earth itself. Our ecological peril does so too.

Lifeline represents an attempt to foster the form of love Schell calls generative and others have called preservative (cf. Gray 1970; Ruddick 1984). Whether it is in all respects a satisfactory attempt is not the isssue here. The point to be made is that generative love has to be learned: it is not something "innate" that we can count on emerging automatically as people mature. Moreover, today's startling statistics on child abuse, rape, and family violence testify that this love will not necessarily be acquired informally in the course of growing up, at least not in our society. If a new form of love is what the future requires, we must look to education. The anomalous status of *Lifeline* is symptomatic, however, of the precarious position of any approach to education that focuses on generative love and the ethics of care this involves. Examine the recent national reports on education in the United States (e.g., Adler, 1982; Boyer 1983; Goodlad 1984; Sizer 1984). You will find repeated demands for proficiency in the three Rs, for clear, logical thinking, and for higher standards of achievement in science, mathematics, history, literature. You will search in vain, however, for discussions of or recommendations regarding love. Why are there no calls for mastery of the three Cs of care, concern, and connection? To answer this question is to understand why *Lifeline* is anomalous and why the neglect of moral sentiments by other models of moral education is viewed with equanimity.

THE CONTEMPORARY IDEAL OF THE EDUCATED PERSON

On one level the answer to our question is simple. Assuming that the "true" object of education is the development of mind, we subscribe to an ideal of the educated person that gives pride of place to intellectual virtues and attainments. Couldn't education develop intellectual virtues and also the feelings, emotions, values, and attitudes the future requires? Of course it could, but our current assumptions about the function of education do not allow us to conceive of the educated person in this inclusive way. Let me explain.

In the late twentieth-century United States—if not in all times and places—the educated person is one who has had, and profited from, a liberal education.[1] He or she will have been initiated into the various forms of knowledge and will have acquired, along with a body of information, conceptual schemes and cognitive perspectives by which to interpret experience (Peters 1972). Educators and philosophers argue over the exact number of forms of knowledge: Are there seven, nine or five? They disagree about how to distinguish them: Are physics and biology separate forms or not? They debate the qualifications of specific candidates: Is art a form of knowledge at all? Is religion? There is, however, remarkable consensus about the broad outlines, if not the specific details, of both liberal education and our overarching ideal of the educated person. It is generally accepted that the object of liberal education is to develop mind, that a well-developed mind is governed by reason, that rational mind is defined as the acquisition of knowledge and understanding, and that the preferred kind of knowledge is theoretical.

Needless to say, in defining the educated person as one possessing rational mind and construing this latter in intellectualistic terms, feelings and emotions and other so-called "noncognitive" states and processes of the individual are all but ignored. Except for the skills and procedures required in order to use the conceptual schemes of the disciplines in interpreting the world, procedural knowledge—*knowledge how* as philosophers sometimes call it—is neglected, too. What is perhaps less apparent, but equally important, is that this ideal also makes suspect the development of physical capacities, artistic talents, and effective moral action.

The great irony of liberal education today is that it is neither tolerant nor generous. The liberally educated person—which is to say, the educated person—will have knowledge about others but will not have been taught to care about their welfare. That person will have some understanding of society but will not have been taught to feel its injustices or even be concerned about its fate. Our educated person is an ivory tower person: one who can reason but has no desire to solve real problems in the real world; one who understands science but does not worry about the uses to which it is put; one who can reach flawless moral conclusions but has neither the sensitivity nor the skill to carry them out effectively. Alternatively, he or she is a technological person: one who wants to solve real-life problems and has the requisite skills but cares nothing about the real-life consequences of solutions to them.

John Dewey devoted his life to combatting the tendency to separate reason from emotion, thought from action, education from life. Nevertheless, the dualisms he tried to lay to rest continue to haunt us. The distinction we draw between liberal and vocational education represents a separation of mind from body, head from hand, thought from action. In identifying "true" education with liberal, not vocational, study, we build this cluster of splits into our ideal. Because we equate educated persons with educated minds and interpret the concept of mind narrowly, a split between reason and emotion is built into our ideal also. But this is not all. Valuing rationality for its contributions to self-control and personal autonomy, we embrace an ideal that cuts the self off from others. No intimations of human connectedness complicate the picture. The ability to sustain human relationships, a desire to care for and nurture other living beings, a sense of oneness with nature—these are not considered relevant. The ideal guiding education today divorces self from other even as it alienates each separate self from its own body and emotions.

Where does this lopsided ideal come from? Why does it hold us in thrall? The first party I introduced into the conversational circle I constructed in my book *Reclaiming a Conversation* (1985) was Plato. I began with him there and invoke his name now because the ideal I have just described has its roots in the *Republic*. Once adjustments are made for Plato's antidemocratic politics and his distrust of empirical knowledge, one can see that our contemporary conception of the educated person is patterned on the ideal he constructs to guide the education of the guardians of his Just State.

Because Plato takes ruling to be a matter of knowing The Good and considers this knowledge to be the most abstract kind there is, he requires the rulers of the Just State to engage in rigorous theoretical study so as to perfect their deductive powers and develop the qualities of objectivity and emotional distance. To be sure, not one of Plato's guardians will be the "disembodied mind" sanctioned by our own ideal, for Plato believed that a strong mind requires a strong body. Nonetheless, he designed for his rulers an education of heads, not hands. Moreover, considering the passions to be unruly and untrustworthy, Plato held up for the guardians an ideal of self-discipline and self-government in which reason keeps feeling and emotion under tight control. As a consequence, although he wanted the guardians to be so connected to one another that they would feel each other's pains and pleasures, the educational ideal he developed emphasized "inner" harmony at the expense of "outward" connection.

THE FUNCTION OF EDUCATION RECONSIDERED

The qualities and traits Plato incorporated into the ideal governing the guardian education and which we incorporate into our ideal of the educated person are ones our society associates with males.[2] According to our cultural stereotypes, men are objective, analytical, rational, interested in ideas and things. They are not interpersonally oriented; they are neither nurturant nor supportive, empathetic nor sensitive. According to our stereotypes, feeling and emotion, nurturance and supportiveness, empathy and sensitivity are female attributes (Kaplan and Bean 1976; Kaplan and Sedney 1980). Why should our overarching educational ideal be limited in this way? Is it simply that we value so-called "masculine" traits more than so-called "feminine" ones? It is more than this. The function we assign education makes the neglect of so-called feminine qualities and traits seem a necessity.

In my research on the place of women in educational thought I have invoked a distinction between the productive and the reproductive processes of society and have argued that both in and outside the academy those concerned with education define the educational realm in relation to society's productive processes, not its reproductive ones. Briefly, the reproductive processes include not simply the biological reproduction of the species, but the rearing of children to maturity and the related activities of managing a household, caring for the sick and elderly, and serving the needs and purposes of family members. In turn, the productive processes include political, social, and cultural activities as well as economic ones. This distinction is related to the one often drawn between the public and private spheres or realms, for in our society reproductive processes are for the most part carried on in the private world of the home and domesticity, and productive processes in the public world of politics and work.

Needless to say, the educated person of our ideal is not taught to carry on all productive processes of society. Aiming at the development of rational mind, a liberal education prepares one to be a consumer and creator of ideas, not an auto mechanic or factory worker. A vocational education prepares one to work with one's hands and use procedures designed by others. These are very different kinds of education, yet both are intended to fit students to carry on only productive societal processes.

I stress our cultural definition of education as preparation for carrying on the productive processes of society because in our culture the private world and its associated processes is thought to be the natural location of feeling and emotion, intimacy and connection, and hence a realm of the nonrational. In contrast, the public world and its associated processes is considered the realm of the rational. Feeling and emotion have no place in it, and neither do intimacy and connection. Instead, analysis, critical thinking, and self-sufficiency are the dominant values. It is to be expected, then, that the development of feeling and emotion, intimacy and connection is ignored by education, whether liberal or vocational. Since we take the function of education to be that of equipping people to carry on well society's productive processes, from a practical standpoint would it not be foolhardy for it to foster these traits?

Only in light of the fact that education turns its back on the reproductive processes of society can the anomalous status of *Lifeline* be understood. As we currently define education, there is no place in our ideal of the educated person, hence no place in moral education, for the love and caring *Lifeline* wants its students to learn. In our culture love and caring are not only linked to the reproductive processes of society, they are thought to be dysfunctional in relation to society's productive processes. Thus, to override the theoretical and practical grounds for ignoring them, the reproductive processes of society will have to be brought into the educational realm and education will have to be defined in relation to *both* kinds of societal processes.

All of us—male and female—participate in the reproductive processes of society. In the past, many have thought that education for carrying them on was not necessary. These processes were assumed to be the responsibility of women and it was supposed that by instinct a woman would automatically acquire the traits and qualities associated with them. The contemporary statistics on child abuse are enough by themselves to put to rest the doctrine of maternal instinct. Furthermore, both sexes have responsibility for making the reproductive processes of society work well. Family living and childrearing are not today, if they ever were, solely in the hands of women. Nor should they be. Thus, both sexes need to learn to carry on the reproductive processes of society just as in the 1980s both sexes need to learn to carry on the productive ones.

Although the reproductive processes are of central importance to society, it would be a terrible mistake to suppose that the traits and qualities traditionally associated with them have no relevance beyond them. On the contrary, today there is every reason to believe that they have the broadest moral, social, and political significance; that care, concern, connectedness, nurturance are as important for carrying on society's economic, political, and societal processes as its reproductive ones.

TRANSACTIONS OF GENDER

If education is to help us acquire generative love, it must be redefined. Once redefined, *Lifeline* will not be the anomaly it now is. The required redefinition of education is not easily accomplished, however. Just as traits and qualities are gender related, so are the two kinds of societal processes: historically, in our culture males have been given primary responsibility for performing the productive processes and females the reproductive ones. It is no accident that our ideal of the educated person coincides with our cultural stereotype of a male human being. Indeed, it could hardly be otherwise. For insofar as education is viewed as preparation for carrying on processes historically associated with males, it can be expected to inculcate traits the culture considers masculine.[3]

Our societal processes and their associated traits are gender related and education is gender related, too. Our definition of its function makes it so. Of course, it is possible for members of one sex to acquire personal traits or qualities our cultural stereotypes attribute to the other. Thus, females can and do acquire traits incorporated in our educational ideal. However, these traits are *genderized*; that is, they are appraised differently when they are possessed by males and females (Beardsley 1977). For example, whereas a male will be admired for his rational powers, a woman who is analytical and critical will be derided or shunned or will be told that she thinks like a man. Even if this latter is intended as a compliment, because we take masculinity and femininity to lie at opposite ends of a single continuum, she will thereby be judged as lacking in femininity and, as a consequence, judged abnormal or unnatural. Similarly, although a female will be praised for her daintiness, a male will be judged effeminate and scorned for possessing this characteristic. Elizabeth Janeway (1971 p. 96) has said, and I am afraid she is right, that "unnatural" and "abnormal" are the equivalent for our age of what "damned" meant to our ancestors.

When those born female are educated, as they are now, in so-called "masculine" traits for which they are denigrated, this negative evaluation reverberates in the way and the extent to which the traits are acquired. Were education to be defined so as to give the reproductive processes of society their due; were nurturing capacities and the three Cs of care, concern, and connection incorporated into the ideal governing the education of both sexes; educated men could be expected to suffer for possessing traits genderized in favor of females as educated women now do for possessing traits genderized in favor of males. This is not to say that males would be placed in the double bind educated females find themselves in now, for males would acquire traits genderized in their own favor as well as ones genderized in favor of females, whereas the traits educated females must acquire today are all genderized in favor of males. On the other hand, since traits genderized in favor of females are considered lesser virtues, if virtues at all (Blum 1980), and the societal processes with which they are associated are thought to be relatively unimportant, males would be placed in the position of having to acquire traits both they and their society considered inferior.

One of the most important findings of contemporary scholarship on women is that our culture embraces a hierarchy of values that places the productive processes of society and their associated traits above society's reproductive processes and the associated traits of care and nurturance. There is nothing new about this. We are the inheritors of a tradition of Western thought according to which the functions, tasks, and traits associated with females are deemed less valuable than those associated with males. In view of these findings, the difficulties facing those of us who would transform moral education in the manner the future requires become apparent.

The magnitude of the changes to be wrought by an education that takes generative love seriously must be understood. Granted, when girls today become educated, they acquire traits genderized in favor of the "opposite" sex. However, they can at least console themselves that their newly acquired traits, along with the societal processes to which these traits are attached, are considered valuable. Were we to attempt to change the nature of our educational ideal without also changing our society's value hierarchy, boys and men would have no such consolation. Yet without this consolation, we can be quite sure that the change we desire will not come to pass. One cannot expect people to endorse an education in traits and qualities they consider suspect.

The film *Yentl* starkly portrayed the human cost of our stereotypical conceptions of masculinity and femininity. The girl Yentl almost literally had to become a man to become an educated person. Once educated, she had to remain a man because the cognitive dissonance, to say nothing of the societal disgrace, of being both a woman and rational made it impossible for her to be accepted as a normal human being. Through schooling and higher education we are well on our way to detaching rationality from masculinity and making it a "normal" attribute of both sexes, although by no means is that journey over. To achieve our future we must embark on the equally difficult—possibly much more hazardous—journey of detaching generative love from femininity so that it, too, can be a "normal" attribute of both sexes.

Paradoxically, as we move away from our stereotypes it is necessary to pay close attention to gender. For only if we remain aware of the devaluation of women and their associated tasks and traits wherever this occurs—whether in the disciplines of knowledge themselves, our classrooms, the larger educational community or society at large—and do something about it, will we be able to incorporate generative love into our ideal of the educated person. And only if we build into our courses of study an examination of gender and the ways our stereotypes function to keep men as well as women in their "places," will generative love be perceived as a possession worth having.

THE ADDITIVE HYPOTHESIS

Suppose now that we succeed in bringing the reproductive processes of society into the educational realm and in defining education in relation to them as well as to society's productive processes. And suppose we incorporate generative love and its three Cs of care, concern, and connection in our ideal of the educated person. What implications would this reconceptualization of our most fundamental assumptions about education have for moral education? Granted, *Lifeline* would no longer be an anomaly. There would most likely be a proliferation of approaches focusing on moral sentiments. But in what relation would approaches such as *Lifeline* stand to models of moral education that focus on moral reasoning, as most now do?

It is tempting to suppose that the relation would be additive. After all, to bring generative love into our overarching educational ideal is not to exclude reason from it. To be sure, our present philosophy of education divorces reason from feeling and emotion in general, and from moral sentiments in particular. According to our stereotypical conceptions of the two kinds of societal processes, only the reproductive ones require generative love in order to be performed well; moreover, because they do, they are considered nonrational, if not irrational human activities. Nevertheless, generative love's goals of protection and growth (cf. Gray 1970; Mayeroff 1971; Noddings 1984; Ruddick 1984) can only be satisfied if intelligence is brought into the service of care, concern, and connection.

To suppose that if our object is to foster generative love we cannot foster moral reasoning is to fall prey to one of the many false dilemmas that continues to victimize educational theory and philosophy. It is, indeed, to endorse the self-same dichotomy that now leads moral educators to assume that because they aim at developing moral reasoning, they must not dwell on the acquisition of moral sentiments. Yet the fact that generative love is compatible with reason does not automatically lend support to the hypothesis that we could hold onto the programs in moral reasoning we already have and simply introduce ones in generative love as a kind of supplement to them. Attractive as this additive vision may be in its ease of implementation, the conception of moral reasoning that lies at the heart of many contemporary approaches to moral education militates against it.

The philosopher H. L. A. Hart has suggested that the study of law has much to teach us about morality. He might have added that it can teach us about moral education as well. In many, perhaps most, approaches to moral education today, morality is viewed as a matter of making moral decisions and these, in turn, are conceived of as judgments or conclusions of impartial, objective individuals who weigh the evidence and bring relevant principles to bear. The mode of reasoning of a judge in our legal system serves, then, as the model for the moral reasoning these programs aim to develop. Just as a judge is expected to be objective and impartial throughout the legal proceedings, so the student must learn to display these qualities while making moral decisions. Just as a judge is assumed to be an external observer to the disputes under consideration, not a participant in them, the student must learn to view cases of moral conflict from the outside.

From the standpoint of the educational objective of generative love, this judging model of moral reasoning poses significant problems. Whereas the basis of generative love lies in our connectedness to others, a judge is required to maintain distance. Disconnection, not connection, is the norm. Whereas in generative love one's feelings and emotions are engaged, a judge is required to put these to one side. The absence of sentiment, not its presence, is the norm. Of course, judging could be different: a judge *could* be one who cared for and felt connected to the people in the situations at issue; indeed, a judge *could* nurture growth and development. In our culture and our legal system, however, judging involves the denial of the very qualities generative love affirms.[4]

Requiring the suspension of generative love on the part of those inclined to it, the moral reasoning at which so many approaches to moral education aim presents a clear obstacle to the development of generative love on the part of those who have not yet acquired it. Moreover, in their emphasis on the centrality to moral decision making of distance and separation, these programs implicitly send the message that the three Cs have little, if anything, to do with serious morality. Thus, to embrace the additive hypothesis and adopt the strategy of introducing programs that focus on generative love alongside existing ones that focus on moral reasoning would be to work at cross purposes.

Of course, having incorporated generative love into our guiding educational ideal it would be possible to continue to divide life into two realms or two sets of societal processes and to assign generative love to the one and moral reasoning according to the judging model to the other. Were such a division tenable, an additive strategy might be acceptable. But it is not tenable for many reasons, the most pressing and immediately relevant of which is that the future requires that generative love be exhibited in all areas of life and all societal processes.

A TRANSFORMED LANDSCAPE

Scholars in a wide range of disciplines have discovered that a simple additive solution to the "problem" of the inclusion of women in their subject matter will not work. An additive solution to the problem of the inclusion in moral education of the generative love associated with women will not work either. If moral educators are to give generative love its due, approaches that make judging their model of moral reasoning will have to be abandoned. As I hope I have made clear, generative love requires the exercise of intelligence and the use of reason. Thus, in casting doubt on the use of judging as the paradigm of moral reasoning, I am not questioning the importance of teaching reasoning in programs of moral education. There are many varieties of thinking and reasoning, however. One challenge to be met by moral educators intent on designing the kind of programs the future requires is that of replacing the judging model with modes of thinking and reasoning that serve, support, and enhance generative love.

This challenge confronts moral philosophers and psychologists as well as moral educators. But if the latter group is not alone in having to reconceptualize moral reasoning, it should not suppose that its own responsibility for effecting the needed transformation is therefore diminished or that its own tasks are dependent on the achievements of the academicians. To postpone the transformative task until psychological and philosophical clarity is achieved is to place the future at risk. Moreover, so far as the project of constructing new, transformed approaches to moral education is concerned, postponement is an unnecessary tactic. We are so accustomed to being told that the structure and nature of knowledge determines the school curriculum that we forget that the concerns of education far outrun the theories and conceptual frameworks of the intellectual disciplines (Martin 1970).

I do not want to give the impression, however, that when moral educators take generative love seriously, a replacement of the judging model with some other form of reasoning is the only transformation we can anticipate. As I have already suggested, programs of moral education tend to be reductionist. Morality is equated with decision making, decision making is then viewed as reasoning, and reasoning is conceived of as judging, with dilemmas or conflict situations assumed to be the proper object of that activity. In light of our contemporary ideal of the educated person and our theory of liberal education, this reductive sequence is to be expected. The inclusion in our ideal of generative love raises questions about its validity, however. Requiring us to reject the divorce of reason from feeling and emotion implicit in the judging model, this new objective mandates also a denial of the split between thought and action entailed by the equation of morality with a narrowly defined reasoning.[5] In addition, it forces us to reconsider the central role most programs now assign to individual decision making and choice and to conflict.

That conflict looms large in programs of moral education is not surprising: disputes between opposing parties to controversies are what judging is all about.[6] It is not at all obvious, however, that conflict and controversy are what morality is all about. In daily living moral dilemmas are the exception not the rule. I do not mean to say that we never confront them. Of course we do.[7] But moral life is not reducible to a series of dilemmas nor is it comprised mainly of them. Neither is the resolution of conflict—whether between opposing parties to a dispute, between one's own desires and moral principles, or between competing principles—the only, or even the most, important element of moral thought and action.

Interestingly enough, as ways to cooperate and to maintain connection take clear shape as educational objectives, the aims of solving dilemmas and resolving controversies recede into the background. With the emergence in the foreground of cooperation and connection, individual decision making and choice recede, too. But this is to say that an emphasis on generative love transforms the entire landscape of moral education. And so it must, for this new emphasis requires that we shed many of our most fundamental assumptions about moral education.

The broad contours and configurations of the new landscape have still to be mapped and its many details filled in. In this chapter I have sketched a few of the changes in moral education we can expect to result from the shift in perspective an emphasis on generative love entails. A detailed study of the *Lifeline* curriculum might well suggest others. And the work on women's moral development by Carol Gilligan (1982), on caring by Milton Mayeroff (1971) and Nel Noddings (1984), on maternal thinking by Sara Ruddick (1984; 1985) will surely suggest more. It remains for moral educators, then, to work out the implications of what turns out to be a radical shift in perspective and also to make clear the differences between it and the one most of us now share. This latter task is important because without that comparison firmly in mind, it will be all too easy to take the line of least resistance. In the name of the future, we must withstand the temptation to settle for an additive strategy when introducing generative love into moral education instead of the transformative one the future requires.

NOTES

1. This section of the chapter closely follows Martin (1986). Its thesis was first developed in Martin (1981a).
2. For further discussion of this topic in relation to Plato see Martin (1985, Ch. 2; 1986).
3. The thesis of this section was first presented in Martin (1981b) and was further developed in Martin (1985; 1986).

4. It should be noted that in our culture judging in nonlegal contexts may in fact be different. At least it is not at all obvious that judging as connoisseurship—e.g., the judging of fine wines or violins—involves the distance and separation that judging in our legal system does.
5. See Fred Newmann (1975; cf. Hersh et al. 1980, Ch. 8) for an approach to moral education that rejects this split.
6. Although an emphasis on conflict is part of the judging model of moral reasoning, conflict is detachable from it. Thus, to reject the judging model is not necessarily to deny conflict the major role it now plays in moral education.
7. For an excellent discussion of moral dilemmas see Nussbaum (1986).

REFERENCES

Adler, M. J. (1982). *The Paideia proposal*. New York: Macmillan.

Beardsley, E. (1977). Traits and genderization. In *Feminism and philosophy*, ed. F. A. Elliston, J. English, and M. Vetterling-Braggin. Totowa, N.J.: Littlefield, Adams.

Blum, L. (1980). *Friendship, altruism, and morality*. London: Routledge and Kegan Paul.

Boyer, E. L. (1983). *High School*. New York: Harper & Row.

Gilligan, C. (1982). *In a different voice: Psychological theory and women's development*. Cambridge: Harvard University Press.

Goodlad, J. I. (1984). *A place called school*. New York: McGraw Hill.

Gray, J. G. (1970). *The warrior*. New York: Harper & Row.

Hersh, R. H., Miller, J. P., and Fielding, G. D. (1980). *Models of moral education*. New York: Longman.

Janeway, E. (1971). *Man's world, woman's place*. New York: Morrow.

Kaplan, A. G., and Bean, J. P., eds. (1976). *Beyond sex role stereotypes*. Boston: Little, Brown.

Kaplan, A. G., and Sedney, M. A. (1980). *Psychology and sex roles*. Boston: Little, Brown.

Kohlberg, L. (1973). *Collected papers on moral development and moral education*. Cambridge: Harvard Graduate School of Education.

Martin, J. R. (1970). The discipline and the curriculum. In *Readings in the philosophy of education*, ed. J. R. Martin. Boston: Allyn & Bacon.

_____ . (1981a). Needed: A paradigm for liberal education. In *Philosophy and education*, ed. J. Soltis. Chicago: National Society for the Study of Education.

_____ . (1981b). The ideal of the educated person. *Educational theory* 31: 97–109.

_____ . (1985). *Reclaiming a conversation*. New Haven: Yale University Press.

_____ . (1986). Redefining the educated person: Rethinking the significance of gender, *Educational Researcher* 6: 6–10.

Mayeroff, M. (1971). *On caring*. New York: Harper & Row.

McPhail, P., Ungoed-Thomas, J. R., and Chapman, H. (1975). *Lifeline*. Niles, Ill.: Argus Communications.

Newmann, F. (1975). *Education for citizen action: Challenge for secondary curriculum*. Berkeley, Calif.: McCutchan.

Noddings, N. (1984). *Caring: A feminine approach to ethics and moral education.* Berkeley: University of California Press.

Nussbaum, M. C. (1986). *The fragility of goodness.* Cambridge: Cambridge University Press.

Peters, R. S. (1972). Education and the educated man. In *Education and the development of reason*, ed. R. F. Dearden, P. H. Hirst, and R. S. Peters. London: Routledge & Kegan Paul.

Ruddick, S. (1984). Maternal thinking. In *Mothering*, ed. J. Trebilcot. Totowa, N.J.: Rowman & Allenheld.

––––––– . (1985). Maternal work and the practice of peace. *Journal of Education* 167: 3, 97–111.

Schell, J. (1982). *The fate of the earth.* New York: Avon.

Shaver, J., and Strong, J. (1976). *Facing value decisions: Rationale building for teachers.* Belmont, Calif.: Wadsworth.

Sizer, T. (1984). *Horace's compromise.* Boston: Houghton Mifflin.

11

The Just Community Educational Program: The Development of Moral Role-taking as the Expression of Justice and Care

Ann Higgins

> It's caring and speaking up or saying what I think, without saying what I think or without caring, I wouldn't be me. I mean I can't have caring without speaking up and I can't have speaking up without caring. I need both of them to be me. If I can't have that then I'm not me, I'm acting like somebody else.
>
> 17-year-old woman from
> the South Bronx, 1986

I will begin this chapter by suggesting a practical proposition that justice and care are indivisible insofar as they are moral. While acknowledging that psychological gender differences may exist in approach to self and other, I will raise issues about the adequacy of educational interventions based on those presumed psychological gender differences and give examples from Kohlberg's approach to moral education to illustrate an educational intervention that is consistent with the conception of justice and care as indivisible: the just community approach. I will argue it is consistent with the basic tenets of feminism as a social movement aimed at the elimination of social injustice. I will conclude by arguing that the just community approach promotes the full moral development of the student, male and female, through experiences of moral role-taking.

JUSTICE AND CARE AS INDIVISIBLE

The idea of the unity of justice and care is the idea that care is only known when justice is its context in the activity of human life. I offer a practical example.[1] Consider the following situation: A mother and father have three children. The first-born is given love, care, nurturance, and his developing emotional needs are met. His growing sense of self, competency, and self-esteem are fostered by both his parents. The lives of the other two children are free from any physical and material needs, however the parents are insensitive of their emotional well-being and do little to foster their growing sense of self, competency, and self-esteem.

Would we fault these parents? Would we say they are acting unfairly? Yes, we would at least say that. Would we also say that they are not acting in a caring way? Yes, most of us would likely say that. We might try to justify the differential treatment of the children by saying that the oldest boy is more sensitive, brighter, more cooperative etc. However, such justifications would find their limit. We would not say that the differential treatment that exists is right or good or that it is moral.

What if the parents openly admitted that they loved the oldest child the most and, therefore, found it difficult to act as lovingly toward or to be as interested in the others' development and well-being. Would we say that their feelings are a moral or legitimate basis for different treatment of their children? No. We would encourage them to see their other children in such a way as would generate in them the same feelings as they have for their first-born.

If the different treatment continued, we would conclude that the love of the parents for their first-born was unbridled, unmoderated by moral concerns, and label it favoritism, thus redefining the virtue of love as a vice. The care shown the son becomes redefined as expressing some psychological, amoral or immoral, need of the parents. It loses its definition of care altogether.

This illustrates (but does not prove philosophically) the following points. First, that we know care only in the context of justice. The injustice or inequity of this situation propels us to look for explanations of the parents' behavior that lie outside the domain of caring. Care, outside of justice, is not understood in a commonsense way as moral. Therefore, in order for care to be what we know and feel it is, it must be equitable and just. This leads to the philosophical proposition that care, as a moral concept, must be derivable from the idea of justice insofar as it includes the ideas of universalizability and distribution.

Second, and more problematic, is the relation between love, or feelings of love, and care as activity. We recognize and allow for feelings of love to be felt toward some people and not others. We recognize that often parents may feel more love for one child than another. And we recognize that they may not be able to change or control these different feelings. However, we do not consider such feelings as an adequately legitimate or moral basis for caring for children. Our moral expectation is that parents will care for all their children equitably, regardless of their feelings of love. In other words, we expect parents to overcome biases based on feelings of love and to act morally with caring toward all their chilren despite their feelings and preferences.

Thus, love as the basis for the activity of care is inadequate when love is defined only as positive feelings one has toward another. These feelings of love must be combined with higher order empathy or role-taking to become the moral basis of care in action.

Much has been written about love and the various kinds of love. Love as moral activity is usually called by other names—agape, charity, benevolence or mercy. In this chapter I suggest moral role-taking is the social and psychological experience which is the basis for the development of feelings of love as agape, charity, benevolence or what we have written about as community responsibility and valuing (Higgins, Power, and Kohlberg 1984). I suggest that actively practicing moral role-taking engenders within people the experience of themselves as moral beings, able to do both what is right and what is good toward others. This budding idea of the moral self is one focus of our empirical research in the Bronx Just Community educational intervention project. It is through the elaboration of this idea that the indivisibility of justice and care as moral activity will become apparent. The idea of the moral self as necessarily both just and caring is expressed by the 17-year-old woman quoted at the beginning of this chapter.

To address the concern of the relation of justice and care as a psychological area of inquiry, I wish to emphasize the agreement between psychologists who study the development of moral reasoning and those who study the development of moral feelings or empathy. Based primarily on the theories of Piaget and Kohlberg, social scientists who have studied the process by which people develop the capacity for moral reasoning posit, and research studies confirm (e.g., Selman 1980; Walker 1978) that role-taking or taking the perspective of the other is a critical aspect of moral reasoning development. Likewise, psychologists who study empathy and sympathy and their development in children and over the lifespan also find that perspective-taking is central to the full development of these feelings or dispositions (e.g. Hoffman 1979; Eisenberg 1986). This common idea, the development of perspective-taking, cuts across the differences cited by those who put forth gender-related moral notions (e.g., Chodorow 1978; Gilligan 1982; Lyons 1983).

Instead of emphasizing any possible differences in the development of role-taking or perspective-taking due to differences in the development of a sense of identity in girls and boys, I first want to emphasize that both boys and girls do learn to take the view of the other. This, I think puts the cart behind the horse where it belongs. In order to understand differences among people in their moral actions, we first need to understand and agree on some common underlying concepts. Then we may attend to if and how they are manifest in different experiences for females and males which might lead to different conceptions of the self, of morality, and of the world.

Understanding common underlying processes in the development of the moral person is a practical necessity as well. It is necessary in order to have an adequate basis for a theory of moral education for all people. It is a practical necessity for a second reason also, a reason that runs parallel with a definition of feminism as a social movement rather than as an ideology, philosophy or psychology. Human beings are weak creatures given to prejudice and ethnocentrism. We have created imperfect social structures which express our sense of community with others but which as well express our suspicions, alienation, and power-grasping. For us to become moral individuals and moral communities and societies we must attack prejudice and the misplacement and misuse of power at two levels simultaneously, the level of individual change and of social change. Feminism as a social movement demanding the elimination of injustice is aimed at the second level. Developing more education programs in which girls and boys alike learn to respect others, see and emphasize with other points of view, and fully consider the others in arriving at a solution or conclusion is creating justice and care at the individual level.

At this time in the development of ourselves and our cultures it seems very difficult for us to emphasize differences and to maintain equal and equitable treatment of individuals and of groups. To highlight or glorify differences now leads quickly to stereotyping, assigning people to categories, and to misinterpretation of the individual's life and talents in terms of the range of talents average or common to that sex, race, ethnic group or social class. As an example consider the diverse reactions of white people to the Black Power/Pride movement during the 1960s and 1970s in the United States. Many of the reactions were based on dualistic stereotypes of black people. In Chapter 3 of this book Toinette Eugene chronicles the fight of black women in the United States against the dehumanizing institution and practices of slavery and its aftermath, describes the demoralizing stereotype of the black woman held by whites, and recounts the rich complexity of the black woman's view of herself and of her place in black culture and in American culture. The vast and layered reality of black women may not have been fully expressed in the Black Power/Pride movement but the reactions of whites in terms of simple stereotypes showed us to be ignorant of the realities of black people, and especially black women. In contrast, regardless of their attitudes and beliefs, white people have been legally required by our society's view of what is morally right and just to acknowledge the civil rights movement and to support the efforts of this movement by upholding new laws passed to eliminate areas of prejudicial treatment. I do not intend to speak against black pride or the pride of any group or to gloss over differences among human beings or cultures; however, I do want to make the point that the discovery and fight for full recognition of possible differences among us should take place on the bedrock of justice and the recognition of our common humanity, fundamental aspects we still must struggle to manifest in our lives together.

A DEFINITION OF FEMINISM AS SOCIAL POLICY

In *The Sceptical Feminist* Janet Radcliffe Richards (1980) argues that feminism should not be concerned with women "per se" but should rather be concerned with "a type of injustice it wants to eliminate: the injustice which women suffer as a result of being female" (p. 271). Moreover, Richards argues that in this current era "Things are made systematically harder for women than for men in the same position and with identical abilities. Women are discriminated against" (Richards 1980, p. 272) and this discrimination is practiced by both individuals and institutions. Richards offers an agenda for the present and future work of feminism: To change and rearrange the structures of institutions in order to foster equality, fairness, and the full development of individuals.

We need not accept that anything which is kept from the past must be kept in its past form. The radical thing to do is to insist on splitting up the packages, by working carefully at what is good and what is bad about the institutions of the past. What is good must be kept wherever possible. It is no business of feminism to go in for a simple reaction against the past; to throw out everything which happens to have male fingerprints on it. To the extent that feminists do this and in doing so deprive everyone of the good things which might have been possible if they had been more imaginative, they are directly allowing the past to cause trouble in the future. They have failed in radicalism, and through a lack of care in working things out have set out on a path which leads to precisely the opposite of the good they were trying to achieve (Richards 1980, p. 290).

I propose in this chapter that the just community is such a radical rearrangement of educational structures. Thus, it promotes the full development of all its students. Before describing why the just community approach is a good way for promoting the full development of students I want to summarize two other streams of moral education and their limitations: character education and values clarification. Many femininists interested in reforming educational practices to enhance sexual equality and include feminine virtues have implicitly and perhaps unknowingly rested their arguments upon the assumptions of one of these two approaches. Since I think the value assumptions of these approaches lead to the creation of limited and not truly transforming educational practices, I wish to persuade feminists interested in true educational reform to ground their ideas in moral theories that have the power to transform. I will argue that theories of morality that are based in developmental psychology and that recognize a universal core of moral concerns are more powerful bases for the educational reforms sought by feminists than those based on learning theories of psychology and moral theories of value relativity. The transforming power of the practices of the just community approach lie in its psychological and philosophical assumptions.

FEMINISM, CHARACTER EDUCATION, VALUES CLARIFICATION

With these ideas in mind, let us consider two current approaches to moral education, character education and values clarification. In the 1920s and 1930s and again now in the 1980s, the approach of character education has been widely prevalent in U.S. public schools. The educators and psychologists who developed these approaches defined character as the sum total of a set of "those traits of personality which are subject to the moral sanctions of society" (Havighurst and Taba 1949). For Hartshorne and May (1928) these traits included honesty, service, and self-control. For Havighurst and Taba (1949) they included honesty, loyalty, responsibility, moral courage, and friendliness. These traits are similar to those noted by Aristotle which included temperance, liberality, pride, good temper, truthfulness, and justice, and by those encouraged by the Boy and Girl Scouts—honesty, loyalty, reverence, cleanliness, and bravery.

A main difficulty with this approach is that it is value-relative. The composition of the list of virtues and the priorities given different virtues varies from one theory or practice to another and from one historical era or society to another.

The problem of values relativity in character education approaches has become the virtue of values clarification approaches. In more recent U.S. history, values clarification approaches have emerged as a response to the recognition that our society is a complex association of various ethnic and racial groups holding diverse values and living within social institutions with various normative structures. This value-relative approach to moral education is consistent with a larger approach to problems of diversity in our society—let each person do his or her own thing.

As summarized by Engel this position holds that "in the consideration of values, there is no single correct answer, but value clarification is supremely important" (Simon, Howe, and Kirschenbaum, 1972, p. 902). The values clarification approach is widely used and, I think, can be a valuable component of educational curriculums. However, the limitations should be stated. First, values clarification offers no solution to the problem of the relativity of values. Second, the actual teaching of relativism is itself an indoctrination or inculcation, teaching of a fixed belief.

Feminism, as I have defined it here, is incompatible with values clarification and most character education programs. A feminist perspective cannot accept the assumption that values are relative, since feminism holds equality between the sexes as a universal, nonrelative value and the elimination of social injustices due to one's gender as an absolute good. Out of concern for respecting individual rights, values clarification advocates favor the use of rational strategies, which is the focus of systems of procedural justice. However, feminists must maintain that procedural justice alone is an inadequate response to issues of discrimination and prejudice. Problems of social injustice or the violation of individual rights need to be tackled as issues of substantive justice as well. Value clarification approaches allow young sexists, either male or female, to remain stuck in conventional biases while offering the teacher no solid ground, no substantive principles, from which to challenge stereotypical thinking.

Following Richards (1980), I have suggested that feminism's central concern is the elimination of injustices against women due to their sex alone. A character education approach (Havighurst and Taba 1949) which focuses on the content of human character, may or may not have some relation to this primary feminist goal. Such a curriculum defines and shapes virtues and vices; it may explore issues central to feminism, though none of its core assumptions necessitate that exploration. For example, some theorists (Martin 1985, also this volume; Noddings 1984, also this volume) have proposed a new kind of character education. Both Martin and Noddings discuss transforming moral education in the light of what each, although differently, describes as feminine characteristics. Martin speaks of the three Cs: care, concern, and connection, as traits genderized in favor of females, which ought to be developed in all students through education. Noddings argues for the incorporation of female experience and the maternal model into the moral education curriculum.

In my opinion, both of these feminist philosophers are seeking a fundamental overhaul of the educational system, something that sharply differentiates them from traditional character education approaches but stops short of the restructuring of the schools that Richards (1980) recommends. I am in agreement with their call for including women's historical and present experience in educational curriculums. I am more hesitant about interpretations of women's experience as exclusive of male experience and am wary of theories (e.g., Chodorow 1978; Rossi 1977) that postulate psychological or biological essentialism to explain the source of gender differences.

Much gender research in education (Tittle 1986; Dweck 1986) has shown that constellations of so-called male and female traits arise out of specific and particular social interactions and situations. They are consequently more complex and variable than much theoretical work indicates. Attempts to create educational programs that seek to teach boys as well as girls the positive "feminine" traits will probably be even less successful than traditional character education programs that seek to teach virtues, supposedly not gender-related, since they will be hindered by the existing sexism in our society. Boys will not value nurturance or compassion any more than they do now for having been required to learn about them. In order to instill the feminine virtues and accomplish the transformation of education espoused by Martin, Noddings, and others, changes in the curriculum must be accompanied by structural changes in the school which will result in the formation of new normative and value structures.

We call the normative and value structures of a school the moral atmosphere or moral culture and seek to create a more just and caring school climate through instituting the structures of the just community program (Power, Higgins, and Kohlberg 1989). A summary of the changes in the school moral climate due to the implementation of a just community program in an inner city school will be reported following a description of the program.

In a recent review of gender research education, Tittle (1986) concluded that gender perceptions and behaviors influence differential educational and occupational outcomes for men and women. She argued that research indicates that these differences are related to the social interactions between peers and with teachers in the school. Among other recommendations, Tittle called for gender-related research in education to focus on studies of the school as a social institution. She emphasized that research is needed to identify those schools and programs which are effective in attaining gender equity. Although we have not systematically studied the effects of the just community approach on teachers' and students' constructions and perceptions of gender roles or gender-related behavior, such an enterprise is of value and is possible. In this chapter, I will illustrate how such research could proceed by giving examples of students' growth in the areas of social perspective-taking and moral role-taking. I will also suggest that the just community is an approach to moral education that in its ideal form exemplifies the feminist goal to eliminate social injustice due to sexism. Both share the moral philosophical assumption of equal respect for the dignity and worth of each person.

THE JUST COMMUNITY APPROACH

In contrast to values clarification and character education, the just community approach exemplifies Richards's (1980) call for a radical restructuring of the educational structure to achieve social justice. Based in cognitive developmental theory, this view of moral education was first fully stated by John Dewey (1959). It is called cognitive because it recognizes that moral education, like intellectual education, has its basis in stimulating the active thinking of the child about moral issues and decisions. It is called developmental because it sees a central aim of moral education as movement through moral stages.

Just community programs have been in existence for over a decade. This approach differs from small-group moral dilemma discussions, in that just community programs attempt to affect the moral atmosphere or climate of a school. The primary goal of this program is to create and provide an environment in which issues of fairness, justice, community, and caring are democratically debated and resolved. Rules are established and enforced through the active participation of all members, teachers and students, each having one vote. We consider the active participation of the students and teachers in such a complex, democratic, rule-governed organization as the appropriate means to enhance the social and moral development of individual students as well as the appropriate means for making the school itself a more caring, fair, and just institution in which to learn and to work (Higgins, Power, and Kohlberg 1984; Power 1980).

This program represents an effort to balance justice and community, to introduce the powerful appeal of the collective while both protecting the rights of the individuals and promoting their moral growth. The justice aspect of the program is embodied in the democratic process through moral discussions that consider issues of fairness, rights, and duties. In an ideal program the students and teachers evolve their own value positions through moral discussion and democratic decision making and translate those individual positions into rules and norms for group behavior. These rules and norms form the basis of the institution. The teachers not only facilitate discussion among students, but also lead them in decision making by advocating, as opposed to coercing or remaining neutral, value positions that they see as in the best interest of the group. The moral advocacy of the teachers must be strictly bounded by the safeguards of democratic process to avoid becoming indoctrination; the democratic process must become an institutionalized structure in order to avoid becoming rule by the subgroup, the strong or the highly verbal.

The community aspect of the program is an attempt to create a more ideal form of society within the school. Here the pragmatic-associational aspects of schooling (attending classes, teaching and learning, keeping order, forming cliques, etc.) are transformed when a 'sense of community' shared by the members is the context in which schooling takes place. Rather than simply school routines that have to be managed, they become shared aspects of communal life. The community aspect is the motivational power of the group which encourages students to act upon their better moral judgments, to translate moral reasoning and feelings into moral action. Thus, community is a call for students and teachers to participate in school in a caring way such that the rules and concerns of the program become personally felt and community-shared responsibilities of and to all members. Community and justice, then, are the main moral content advocated by this approach.

I will now turn to a description of one just community, some initial research results, and quotations from student interviews to describe how community meetings are run, to define the obligations and responsibilities of the community members, and to illustrate the concepts of moral role-taking and the moral self.

In 1985, two just community programs were initiated in New York City schools, with Larry Kohlberg as the primary consultant. One school draws academically high achieving students from all five boroughs, the other school is an inner city, working class and poor neighborhood school in the

Bronx. This second school will be the focus of this discussion. One hundred voluntary members for the just community program were recruited from a student population of 3,000. Almost all of the students in the school are black or Hispanic with some Asians and Native Americans. The majority of the faculty are white and middle class. The school has a high truancy rate; at least one-third of the students do not graduate, and a large proportion of the students is involved with social service agencies in some way.

The entire community of 100 students and four teachers meet for two class periods one day a week; advisory/discussion groups of 25 students and one teacher meet another day; committees meet a third day; and staff meet a fourth day. An academic class combining English, social studies, and moral discussion meets one of the two periods, four days a week. Despite the limited time together, the students and teachers have created a community they value highly.

Initial analyses of moral reasoning data from this just community project (Higgins 1987) show similar upward stage change for these students as is usually found in other moral discussion (Higgins 1980) and just community (Power, Higgins, and Kohlberg 1989) interventions. In both the working class/poor neighborhood school and in the mainly middle-class high achieving magnet school the just community students' moral judgment developed one-quarter stage on average during the first year of the program. Comparison students from the parent high schools showed no moral stage development over the same time period. The more disadvantaged students from the neighborhood school in both the program and comparison groups entered the study reasoning on average at stage 2/3 or at a preconventional level, while both groups of students from the high achieving magnet school began the study reasoning on average at stage 3, the first stage of the conventional level. The fact that the amount of stage change is the same across schools indicates that the just community program is as effective in promoting the major shift from preconventional to conventional reasoning in youth below the average for their age in moral reasoning, as it is for promoting growth in youth reasoning at the age-appropriate conventional level. These results are noteworthy because this is the first study to show that significant moral stage development occurs as a result of a just community experience less than one-half of each school day and with adolescents still reasoning primarily at the preconventional stages.

We think that the restructuring of governance from a hierarchical model found in the parent high schools to the democratic model of the just community creates a shift in students' perceptions of the moral atmosphere or culture of the school. For two years we compared responses to a moral atmosphere questionnaire of students who have been in the just community program with their comparison group peers in the regular high school. We found that the just community students are consistently and significantly more positive about many aspects of the moral culture of their program than the comparison group students are of the moral culture of the high school. Just community students thought their rules were more fair, that they have better relationships with their peers and with teachers, and that they have a stronger sense of community and feeling of pride about their program than do the comparison high school students. Just community students also perceived significantly less fighting and vandalism and more incidents of students helping than did their comparison peers in the regular high school. More importantly, the just community students reported that strong prosocial norms exist in their community—norms of caring for others, listening to others, taking other people's points of view, stopping to think before acting, and learning to speak up or participate. These results show that a radical restructuring of the governance model of a school can create more fair rules and more prosocial norms which are reflected in our measures of the moral atmosphere of a school or program. Elsewhere we have argued that the democratic governance model of the just community embodies the philosophical tenet of equal respect for the dignity of each person (Power, Higgins, and Kohlberg 1989). Here I want to argue more specifically that the experience of democratic self-governance through manifesting this universal principle is a process for eliminating sexism in the schools as Richards (1980) had recommended. To do that I will present excerpts from student interviews recounting how they learned to participate in a democratic community.

Hazel, a black female who grew up in the South and moved to New York as an adolescent, described a working democracy in the community meeting this way.

The chairperson just keeps order and says, "Wait, you can't talk." And he tells who can talk in turn. You know, he is like a peacemaker. When I said everyone helps out before, I mean everybody makes the rules. If I make a motion, everybody who wants to say something on it gets a chance to say, "Wait, I feel this way or I feel that way. This is a bad motion." Somebody else will get a chance to say that "This is the good part of it." If everybody makes a rule it is not like they say, "Well, listen, we made a rule that you are not going to do this and you all are not going to do it no matter what you say." Everybody makes the rules.

Hazel also tells us that it is not all orderliness and polite listening to each other's opinions. There is sometimes chaos, arguing, and even disrespect. However, such instances are the very substance from which we build a community and create a working democratic process. Hazel describes the meeting in which rules against name-calling and walking out of the meeting were established.

Some of the crazy things that people say and the unfairness of it just get you to arguing. It always ends up to be a good meeting; but you argue a lot and there are a lot of "points of order." There was a lot of name calling and a lot of noise, and then afterward

you say, "Wait, what did we accomplish? We accomplished that you can't call people names and you can't get up and walk out of a meeting.

The ideas of mutual respect and treating each other fairly are balanced in
the program by the idea of community, the responsibility of members to
each other and to the group as a whole. Hazel explains her understanding of
each member's responsibility to the community.

A good member of the just community is somebody who comes to the meetings,
somebody who respects everybody in the meetings. They give others a chance to say
what they have to say. But if you're going to be there and be quiet and don't say
anything when a rule is made, and you don't like it, even though when you had the
chance to change it, you didn't, then don't complain. . . . You're responsible to
take part in the meetings and try to help out.

Hazel's description focuses on the responsibility one has to the community, both responsibility for upholding fairness and justice, and responsibility
for building and maintaining relationships. Roberto, an Hispanic youth,
tells how these two aspects of responsibility necessarily give rise to each
other when the structure for moral education is students' public discussion
of moral issues. When asked whether the people of the just community are
different from those in the rest of the high school, he responds:

Well, yes, because even though they [the just community students] might be a little
crazy, they have a sense of unity and responsibility. They're all, a lot of them, are
starting to develop a good sense of moral responsibility. . . . Everybody in there is
responsible for each other and because one wants to speak their mind so badly, it just
comes out, and then, there, you have the trust. You have the trust and the community so you're able to make moral statements. They are developing that and that's what
I think differs them from the rest of the high school.

In interviews with comparison group students from the same high school
we learned that the larger school moral culture was quite negative and
anomic. The comparison students said the norms of the high school are to be
distrustful and unhelpful to all but one's close friends, to expect belongings to
be stolen, and to walk the halls with eyes to the ground so as to avoid giving
offense that might lead to a physical fight. The stated rule most frequently
voiced was "Don't look at somebody wrong or they'll beat you up." In contrast, Hazel and Roberto's descriptions reveal the just community program's
norms of cooperation and responsibility to the group, consistent with the
moral atmosphere questionnaire responses reported above.

MORAL ROLE-TAKING

In a just community program there is also an expectation that members
will actively participate as Hazel and Roberto described. However, this

expectation is based on the assumption that all members *can* participate. That is, all have the necessary verbal and social skills, they are motivated, there is opportunity, and they have the courage and self-esteem necessary to speak in a group of 100 students and teachers. Of course, such is not the case for many students, especially at the beginning of the program. For some, this means learning to discipline oneself to refrain from speaking out, learning to listen to others, and learning to take the other's perspective. This has been a lesson that many of the strongest leaders of the group learned over the first year. For others it means becoming interested, thinking one can offer something to the group, taking one's own opinion as seriously as one takes others' opinions, and finally speaking up, participating actively in a discussion or meeting. One underlying process is involved in both learning to listen and in learning to speak up, the process of a moral role-taking. Moral role-taking is the actual experience of people in a mutually respectful interaction that concludes with a solution felt to be the most morally right or good. It is this experience of moral role-taking that eliminates sexism and other prejudices in members of a just community program (Power, Higgins, and Kohlberg 1989). Moral role-taking is fostered through moral discussion.[2]

Pedro, an Hispanic male, began the program saying that what he wanted from it was "Credit and a couple of girlfriends; to get popular." Pedro has become popular within the just community and the larger high school. He has also learned to take the perspective of others and to listen to others, an outcome he did not anticipate and a task he found difficult for a time. He describes a situation in which he became aware of this new way of relating to people.

I felt that Joe was trying to upstage me, calling me out of order and taking me to the Discipline Committee. But what was I complaining about? I wanted this to happen, to have other people come out of their shells. I think I understand now that he is not trying to upstage me; he just cares and is trying to make the just community work. But I've been a little jealous and now I know the just community doesn't revolve around me.

Clearly for Pedro, the just community is an experience that promoted both moral growth and self-understanding. When he was asked why he chose to run for the student organization presidency, he first spoke of his political ambitions and then of the role the just community program had in his decision to run for office. He begins by saying he wanted the practice.

In order to run for politics. Some of my teachers called me a used car salesman . . . I'm always talking ever since I can remember. I used to be talking out in the classes. I used to get in trouble and all that. The teachers said I didn't have anything to say and probably I didn't have then but now I have something to say . . . A year ago I used to double-talk teachers and stuff, like I would stretch the class and not do the work. I would ask some questions and would spend my time like that. In the just community I would make my mind work and stop talking. Six months ago some of my views changed, I changed my mind in the just community. Now I listen to other people's thoughts. I take some of this and believe some of that and put it together. It's changed my thoughts. I'm listening more to people now.

Pedro is describing the process of change that occurs through democratic discussion: stating an idea, listening to others agree or disagree with it, taking other's perspectives and considering their ideas, modifying one's own, restating it, and listening again. During discussions of issues of fairness and community, strategies of double-talk, asking off-target questions, not thinking, and tuning out dropped dramatically with the students' growing sense that they, with the teachers, must build a positive normative community in order to grow as a group and survive as a program. For Hazel, Pedro, and others building a school community meant they had to take others' perspectives which meant in turn, they had to stop speaking out, listen to others and evaluate their own as well as others' ideas more seriously. This critical component of moral education is moral role-taking, active perspective-taking, and active consideration of others' views. These actions are the essence of respect, of acting out of concern for fairness and care which enables one to make connections with the thoughts, beliefs, and feelings of others in the community.

However, the process of moral education is not the same for all students. Even though they share common experiences and sit in the same democratic community meetings, whether and how they become active participants differs. Here I want to illustrate two kind of students who describe themselves as "quiet." Our observations and the work of other researchers (e.g., Eakins and Eakins 1978) suggest these quiet students are more apt to be girls than boys. For these students the process of moral education is almost the reverse of what I have illustrated with Pedro's responses. These girls articulate movement from feeling like outsiders, to becoming interested, then deciding that they have some responsibility to the group for speaking up at meetings and offering their opinions and, finally, they begin actively to participate.

Maria, an Hispanic student, says her essential quality is her shyness. She offers a behavioral analysis of changes that can be attributed to her being in the just community program. When asked if she is different in the program compared with the large high school, she says she is.

I am very quiet in the just community program. I won't say anything. I listen to what everyone is saying, but I don't give my opinion. The reason I am not saying anything is I won't. I like to hear different views, you know, why you think we should do something that way. I like to hear them out. . . . You should pay attention to what is going on so you won't be a total blank. And you have your own feelings, like if afterwards, if someone asks you what is your opinion on the subject, you know, you have an opinion. You don't lay there like a lump on a log. . . . I don't talk in the big meetings but I talk in the core groups [small advisory/discussion groups of 25 students and one teacher].

Not only is Maria genuinely interested in listening to others, she also considers *that* a responsibility of a good member. However, the rowdy enthusiasm of the large community meetings kept Maria from actively contributing throughout the entire first year (1985). In the fall of 1986, Maria volunteered to speak before a new just community program with 80 ninth-grade repeaters from her high school. Maria chose to speak on overcoming her shyness.

When I joined the just community, we talked about many subjects I knew a lot about. I wish I had the courage then that I have now to raise my hand to express myself, but I sat and watched. I began to realize that if you chair the core group meetings it becomes easier to express your opinion in a large community meeting such as yours. Don't be afraid to speak or express your opinion, what you say no one else may have thought of, you never know; your opinion may be just what the community is looking for.

Maria's sense of responsibility to the just community, supplemented by opportunities to practice in a small group in which she knew everyone, convinced her that being responsible meant adding her unique viewpoint to the discussion; in fact she recognized that this was for the good of the community. Active participation fostered the transformation from fear of being in a spotlight to a desire to be a contributing member of an ongoing discussion. Maria's development is an example of caring or responsible action growing out of her recognition that the community's demand upon her to actively participate was a just demand made in the context of a just group.

The just community approach is defined by the structures of one person, one vote, open and democratic discussion and a conscious attempt to build community, and is based on the assumptions of equality and mutual respect. Thus, it is a program that should have the potential to foster equality and equity among the students who participate in it. Students report this happens in the just community.

Doris, a black girl, describes herself as moody. She feels, and is, somewhat alienated from other students and from the school. She says, "I'm just unpersonable, I don't like to communicate with people." The basis for Doris' view of herself as private and closed is related to her desire to be respected and her perception that she is not. In an interview she defined morality as "respect."

I seldom give respect because I don't get respect. It all depends on the person I'm talking to. If I'm talking to a person that I get the distinct impression that he doesn't respect females, then I'm not going to respect him. But if I'm talking to a person who respects me, then, hey.

The just community is a place where Doris feels that there is mutual respect among members and, therefore, she is willing to speak up, to contribute, and to care for the community group out of respect for its members.

In the just community you have got to respect others. You've got to be a very responsible person. You've got to be mature enough to handle it. In this program that is certainly done. . . . I'm not very talkative, but I can hold a real good conversation if the talking gets real good. If like, for example, I'm in the program, I will stand up in a crowd and address people, otherwise I don't usually do that. I'm basically a quiet person. . . . Being in the just community, I learn to say, "Hey, you can't just sit back, you've got to react." Now I'm doing something. Before I never used to do anything. The just community has helped me that way. You know, people need a little help.

Being in the just community motivated Doris to be more active in school and led her to feel that she belongs to a community whose members respect and help one another.

THE MORAL SELF AND MORAL ACTION

Any program in moral education hopes to change the behavior of the students participating in it. We are concerned that students change their behavior but we are also concerned with why they change and how they understand the changes they make. Theoretically, we think that moral action is the outcome of several variables (see Kohlberg 1984; and Power, Higgins, and Kohlberg 1989 for more complete discussions of this topic): individual moral judgment including one's understanding of his/her obligations, the moral culture of the situation or group, individual will or attention, and one's concept of him/herself as a moral person. Our previous research study of the moral culture of high schools (Higgins, Power, and Kohlberg 1984) argues and illustrates the case that individual moral action is strongly influenced and even determined by the norms and values of the groups of which one is a member. In addition we view a positive moral culture of a group or school as a requirement not only to create the conditions of mutual respect, cooperation, and responsibility among members but for each individual to build a general moral self, a developmental function of the adolescent years.

Here I offer suggestive evidence that one's view of oneself as moral is an important predictor of moral action. Consistent with the theories of Piaget (1965/1932), G. H. Mead (1934), and J. M. Baldwin (1913/1897), we think that the self is constituted through reciprocal interactions with another self but also through interactions with or role membership in a group. We (Kohlberg and Higgins 1987), stress the idea that in adolescence there is the development of a general self related to a "generalized other" (Mead) or an "ideal self" (Baldwin) that is self-consistent or has "character." This general self is primarily constituted by moral rules or principles and as such does not stem from any concrete interaction or group nor is it fully realized in any real group. Rather the general or moral self develops out of the adolescent's active interaction with the group, its rules, norms and values, attempting to shape the group to his/her ideals while simultaneously valuing membership in the group and thus accepting its norms and values, at least in part. This conception of the development of the moral self is parallel to Erikson's idea of identity formation in adolescence. For different reasons, both our symbolic interactionist view and Erikson's psychodynamic view hold that adolescence is the first and prime time for the development of identity or character.

An analysis conducted by Diessner (1988) on a small subsample of 36 students from our research project evaluating the effects of the just community programs in both schools described earlier, focused on the relation of the use of moral terms to describe the self to promise-keeping, a moral action. Students who answered a question about that aspect of themselves they considered to be essential to their sense of self in moral terms were significantly more likely to keep an agreement they had made with our research team to mail back an envelope of completed questionnaires. The students were paid two dollars and asked to promise to return a questionnaire packet within two weeks time. The students who used no moral language in their self-descriptions were significantly less likely to have returned the packets, on time or late. About one-third of the students fit neither extreme, they used some moral language in their initial descriptions but not in answer to the questions asking about their most important or essential characteristics. About one-half of this group returned the packets.

These results, combined with a reading of many student interviews, show us that the students themselves are concerned with the relations among their judgments, feelings, and actions, with being self-consistent or having character—we would say, with developing a moral self.

SUMMARY

The remark quoted at the beginning of this chapter is one young woman's subjective experience of the indivisible nature of justice and care and the necessity of that unity for her self-definition. Through describing our research results and illustrations from student interviews I have tried to lay out the precursors to the development of such a moral self. I have suggested that learning to take another's perspective, a prerequisite for moral judgment development, leads to moral role-taking—listening to and discussing seriously with others in order to make decisions for the good of all and of the whole. Moral role-taking, in turn, fosters the development of a sense of responsibility to care and actively participate, a necessary concomitant to moral action. I have tried to show here that learning to listen, to take another's point of view, to develop a sense of responsibility, and to speak one's thoughts and ideas can be fostered by open democratic discussions within the context of a cohesive community.

More importantly, I have attempted to illustrate that within the just community structures the process of learning is different for different students; yet when equity and equality are norms, all learn to treat one another with respect and care and to participate actively in the community. Finally and most importantly, from a feminist perspective, I have suggested that educational programs which create and explicitly foster the experiences of equality and mutual respect among students and between teachers and students are consistent with the primary goal of feminism: the elimination of social injustices against women and girls due to their sex alone. The just community approach with its structures of democratic community is one program that has genuine potential for realizing this primary goal of feminism.

NOTES

1. A special thank you to Professor Israel Scheffler, Harvard Graduate School of Education, for suggesting this example. Elaborations and inferences are my own responsibility.
2. For excellent workbooks on how to conduct moral dilemma discussions and enhance students' perspective-taking, see Fenton and Gomberg (Gomberg 1980) and Wasserman and Fenton (1982).

REFERENCES

Baldwin, J. M. (1913/1897). *Social and ethical interpretations in mental development*. New York: Macmillan.
Chodorow, N. (1978). *The reproduction of mothering: Psychoanalysis and the sociology of gender*. Berkeley, CA: University of California Press.
Dewey, J. (1959). *Moral principles in education*. New York: Philosophical Library.
Diessner, R. (1988). A constructive developmental view of the moral self in relation to behavior. Ed.D. diss., Harvard Graduate School of Education, Cambridge, MA.
Dweck, C. (1986). Motivational processes affecting successful learning. *American Psychologist* 41: 1,040–48.
Eakins, B., and Eakins, R. (1978). *Sex differences in human communication*. Boston, MA: Houghton Mifflin.
Eisenberg, N. (1986). *Altruistic emotion, cognition, and behavior*. Hillsdale, NJ: Erlbaum and Associates.
Gilligan, C. (1982). *In a different voice*. Cambridge, MA: Harvard University Press.
Gomberg, S. (1980). *An instructor's guide to leading dilemma discussions: A workshop*. Pittsburgh, PA: Carnegie-Mellon University.
Hartshorne, H., and May M. A. (1928–30). *Studies in the nature of character. Volume 1: Studies in deceit. Volume 2: Studies in self-control. Volume 3: Studies in the organization of character*. New York: Macmillan.

Havighurst, J. R., and Taba, H. (1949). *Adolescent character and personality*. New York: Wiley.

Higgins, A. (1980). Research and measurement issues in moral education interventions. In *Moral education: A first generation of research and development*, ed. R. L. Mosher. New York: Praeger.

_____ . (1987). *Year II Report to the W. T. Grant Foundation: An evaluation of the effects of high school democratic governance on student's moral judgment and action*. Graduate School of Education, Harvard University.

Higgins, A., Power, C., and Kohlberg, L. (1984). The relationship of moral atmosphere to judgments of responsibility. In *Morality, moral behavior and moral development*, ed. W. M. Kurtines and J. L. Gewirtz. New York: Wiley.

Hoffman, M. (1979). Development of moral thought, feeling and behavior, *American Psychologist* 34 (10): 958-66.

Kohlberg, L. (1984). *Essays on moral development: Volume II, The psychology of moral development*. San Francisco, CA: Harper and Row.

Kohlberg, L., and Higgins, A. (1987). School democracy and social interaction. In *Social development and social interaction*, ed. W. Kurtines, and J. Gewirtz. New York: Wiley.

Lyons, N. P. (1983). Two perspectives: On self, relationships, and morality. *Harvard Educational Review* 55: 125-45.

Martin, J. R. (1985). *Reclaiming a conversation*. New Haven, CT: Yale University Press.

Mead, G. H. (1934). *Mind, self and society*. Chicago: The University of Chicago Press.

Noddings, N. (1984). *Caring: A feminine approach to ethics and moral education*. Berkeley, CA: University of California Press.

Piaget, J. (1965/1932). *The moral judgment of the child*. Trans. M. Gabain. New York: Free Press.

Power, C. (1980). Evaluating just communities: Towards a method for assessing the moral atmosphere of the schools. In *Evaluating moral development*, ed. L. Kuhmerker, M. Mentkowski, and V. L. Erickson. Schenectady, NY: Character Research Press.

Power, C., Higgins, A., and Kohlberg, L. (1989). *Lawrence Kohlberg's approach to moral education*. New York: Columbia University Press.

Richards, J. R. (1980). *The sceptical feminist: A philosophical enquiry*. London: Routledge and Kegan Paul.

Rossi, A. (1977). A biosocial perspective on parenting. *Daedalus: Journal of the American Academy of Arts and Sciences* 106: 1-31.

Selman, R. L. (1980). *The growth of interpersonal understanding: Developmental and clinical analyses*. New York: Academic Press.

Simon, S. B., Howe, L. W., and Kirschenbaum, H. (1972). *Values clarification*. New York: Hart.

Tittle, C. K. (1986). Gender research and education. *American Psychologist* 41: 1,161-68.

Walker, L. J. (1978). *Cognitive and perspective-taking prerequisites for the development of moral reasoning*. Ph.D. diss., University of Toronto.

Wasserman, E., and Fenton, E. (1982). *The fairness committee manual for high schools*. Cambridge, MA: Cambridge Rindge and Latin High School.

12

Educating Moral People

Nel Noddings

From a feminist perspective, it does not seem credible that the aim of education in current cultures is to produce good people, even though there is much talk about doing exactly that. Indeed, I will argue that a female view reveals that our educational practices have been designed to produce people who, in at least one respect, are *not* good—who are inclined to violence and are unreflective about the ethical codes that support their violent inclinations. I will begin by examining differences between stereotypical masculine and feminine views on good and evil and then argue that analysis and elaboration of an authentic female perspective can contribute greatly to our understanding of moral life. Finally, I will sketch a program for the inclusion of both female and male moral perspectives in the school curriculum, first with respect to developing the good and second with attention to the control of evil.

CONFLICT OVER GOOD AND EVIL

The feminist perspective that I will use has a long history. It has sometimes been called "social" or "maternal" feminism (Black 1983) and has in the past even been identified with a "redemptive" function of motherhood (see Bernard 1975, ch. 18). Its most significant and lasting feature has been an insistence that the logic of women's experience implies a strong stand against violence (Black 1983). Contemporary feminists who have much in common with earlier maternal feminists (which is not to say there are no differences) may be found among both radical feminists (Daly 1984) and psychoanalytic feminists (Dinnerstein 1976; Chodorow 1978). A few present arguments that strongly resemble those of their "maternal" forebears but show considerably more analytic sophistication (Ruddick

1980; 1984). It is a perspective that acknowledges that there are substantial differences between men and women, including differences in their views on moral life. It does not, however, attribute all the differences to biology and nature but traces many of them to centuries of different experience.

In this it differs from the position of the Jungians who attribute differences in male and female assessments of good and evil to differences in essential nature. Because I want to adapt several important insights from Jung and his followers, it is necessary to say at the outset that I reject the Jungian notion of essential, predetermined, and opposite feminine and masculine natures. Some Jungians, for example, go so far as to say that men and women are mirror opposites in their spiritual evaluations. Esther Harding (1976) declares, "That which to man is spiritual, good, and to be sought after, is to woman demonic, powerful, and destructive, and vice versa" (p. 36). This view has done great mischief by locking women and men into values that should be reevaluated as candidates for *human* views of good and evil.

Both women and men have been greatly influenced by stereotypical images of the feminine and masculine. Our society has set its expectations along stereotypical lines. From this perspective, it has been acceptable for women to deplore war and violence and for men to define themselves in various forms of combat. The male view has, however, been dominant and women have been called upon to support the warrior code of honor even though the code represents, for them, a call to evil. When they do not help men to "behave honorably," women are blamed and often blame themselves for what is perceived as moral failure. Harding writes, "The typical story is that he must join his regiment. When he goes to say goodbye to her she coaxes him to remain or is so alluring he forgets his obligation, and the army entrains without him" (1976, p. 81).

But instead of evaluating woman's tendency to put relation before all else as a possible good to be considered by both women and men, as an intuition to be rationally elaborated into a coherent position, Harding claims, "All true women blame the woman who acts in this way, rather than the man. They know that such an action takes unfair advantage of man's vulnerability (1976, p. 81).

This judgment reveals a Jungian belief in the great power of the feminine, but it is here construed as the power of the temptress—the "devil's gateway." Perhaps the most damaging effect of the warrior code on women has been the universal devaluation of virtues thought to be peculiarly feminine. The "law of kindness," for example, is assessed as virtuous so long as it is confined to home and immediate community but is considered evil if it opposes the warrior code (consider the expression "giving aid and comfort to the enemy").

Because they conflict with the warrior code, women's virtues (compassion, responsiveness, tenderness, and the like) have been assessed as weaknesses in public life. Further, weakness itself has long been associated with the "eternal feminine." Paul Ricoeur (1969) speaks of an "eternal feminine" which is more than sex and which might be called the *mediation of the weakness, the* frailty of man" (p. 254). While insisting that this eternal feminine as frailty does not point only at women but at all humankind, he completes his argument with the well-known quotation from *Hamlet*: "Frailty, thy name is woman!" Hence "weakness" and "woman" are synonymous. In many cultures, our own included, it has been, and still is, a terrible insult to call a man "womanish" or to say that he thinks like a woman.

Hatred of feminine attributes has sometimes even induced hatred of religious institutions which represent a component of public life that seems to edify these virtues. Nietzsche, for example, lumped both Christianity and women's thinking together into something he called a "slave mentality." Christian churchmen, he said,

Smash the strong, contaminate great hopes, cast suspicion on joy in beauty, break down everything autocratic, manly, conquering, tyrannical, all the instincts proper to the highest and most successful of the type "man," into uncertainty, remorse of conscience, self-destruction, indeed reverse the whole love of the earthly and of dominion over the earth into hatred of the earth and the earthly (1973 p. 70).

As we shall see shortly, there is much that feminists might agree with in Nietzsche's critique of the church's condemnation of all that is earthly. But Nietzsche has profoundly misinterpreted the church and its real purposes and activities. While it has *preached* what Nietzsche regards as a slave mentality, it has for the most part lived in "autocratic, manly, conquering, tyrannical" ways. With a few significant exceptions, it has remained firmly a part of the warrior mode, and this, from the perspective taken here, is far more evil than a slave mentality.

Outstanding male objectors to the warrior model should be mentioned; these would certainly include Gandhi and Jesus. Each of these men preached nonviolence, loving kindness, and restraint in the pursuit of justice, but each revealed peculiar weaknesses in his private life. Gandhi, for example, seems to have exercised a good bit of psychological violence in his personal life. In his study of Gandhi, Erik Erikson says that he sensed "the presence of a kind of untruth in the very protestation of truth; of something unclean when all the words spelled out an unreal purity; and, above all, of displaced violence where nonviolence was the professed issue" (1969; pp. 230-231). Jesus, while counseling his followers against violence, promised that God would mete out justice in destruction of the wicked. Even his commandment to love one another is ambivalent; in its content, it clearly opposes the warrior code, but in its form—as commandment—it strongly reflects the code. The mother-god might simply say, "I ask you to be gentle with my other children for I love them dearly, too." Recognition of the failure of intimacy that has often accompanied male expressions of universal love and abstract justice is necessary in building an authentic female ethic. In their rejection of physical violence, these men did not completely reject the warrior model: rather, they translated it into a psychological model that still retains power as its goal.

We might, indeed, argue that religious descriptions of evil (constructed by male authorities) have served to mask real evils and even to endorse them. Certainly, they have made women scapegoats for the origin of evil, and the set of myths that accomplished this have demeaned both women and the values they embrace. Mary Daly says of the Adamic myth:

[T]he myth takes on cosmic proportions since the male's viewpoint is metamorphosed into God's viewpoint. It amounts to a cosmic false naming. It misnames the mystery of evil, casting it into the distorted mold of the myth of feminine evil. In this way images and conceptualizations about evil are thrown out of focus and its deepest dimensions are not really confronted (1974, p. 47).

The harm that has been done by the misnaming of evil is incalculable. First, of course, it has inflicted harm on both men and women, but especially on women, by evaluating the earth, body, woman, and nature as lower than heaven, mind, man, and spirit. The devaluation of earth and material interests is one of Nietzsche's great complaints against Christianity, and it is a complaint many feminists share.

Second, it has legitimated the infliction of suffering. Since a God thought to be all-powerful and all-good allows suffering in the world (and even supposedly inflicts it to teach us valuable lessons), human beings have found reasons to justify their own infliction of pain and suffering on each other. For all his opposition to the Christian slave mentality of suffering and sacrifice, Nietzsche—hewing to the warrior model—does not find the infliction or undergoing of suffering objectionable. Rather, he elevates suffering to the status of a criterion for greatness.

Third, because the Augustinian tradition has decreed that the perfection of the universe requires "misery for sinners" (Augustine III, 26), people have projected evil (or sin) onto those whom they would hurt or destroy. Nowhere is this more obvious than in preparation for war, which seems to require almost a frenzy of hatred toward people branded as subhuman, evil, or even monstrous. The need to project evil onto others in order to exteriorize it and thus to destroy it without blaming the self has been turned on women and other "inferiors" as well as on enemies (Daly 1974, p. 76). This point seems to have been especially well understood by Jung and some of his followers (Neumann 1955; von Franz 1983), and I will return to it in the last section.

Fourth, and finally for present purposes, the notion that evil cannot be in God or, by implication, in oneself except insofar as one separates himself or herself from God, leads to a dangerous neglect of what Jungians call our "shadow." If we pretend, for example, that we are all-loving, suppressing our inclinations to hate, we may experience an enantiodromia—a dramatic flow of energy from the pole of love to the pole of hate (Jung 1969). An outburst of violence might be the eventual result. Jung, therefore, suggests that a "morality of evil" (1969, pp. 434, 457) is needed if we are to learn how to control the shadow side. In contrast to Jung's view, which is often considered feminine, Nietzsche—the ultimate masculinist—recommended the incorporation of our devils or shadow in order to become more powerful (see Barrett 1962, pp. 177-205).

In summary, the traditional (masculine) view of evil took the natural association of evil with pain, terror, separation, death, and destruction and transformed it into "ethical terror" (Ricoeur 1969)—fear of transgressing against the patriarch (God, father, church, or state). Thus it misnamed, or covered up, the true nature of evil. In its collaboration with the warrior model, this traditional view may even be accused of participating in evil. Thus there is an analytical task for feminists not only in raising the value of virtues once thought to be feminine but also in redefining and describing evil. Rosemary Radford Ruether says, "Feminism represents a fundamental shift in the valuations of good and evil. It makes a fundamental judgment upon aspects of past descriptions of the nature and etiology of evil as themselves ratifications of evil" (1983, p. 160).

THE NEED FOR A FEMALE PERSPECTIVE

Different outlooks on good and evil lead, logically, to different prescriptions for goodness and for moral education. One would expect considerable overlap in male and female prescriptions as a result of common culture, but because the female view has not been well articulated in the past, mere overlap is often construed as consensus. In part, the lack of articulation is a direct result of the male conception of woman's goodness: silence and service. It is imperative, then, to return to situations that have been analyzed through traditional perspectives and examine them from the viewpoint of women's experience. This involves a reevaluation of both masculine and feminine traits.

In contrast to Harding's judgment that a woman who distracts her lover from duty and honor is "a public menace" (1976, p. 82), we might want to investigate carefully the moral status of such acts and their underlying premises. This is not a simple matter of dismissing a man's obligation to his fellows on the grounds that war is evil in itself; nor is it a matter of declaring women morally justified a priori when they distract men from battle. The proposed program must recognize that there are men who find war glorious, others who defect out of pure self-interest, and still others who go reluctantly but dutifully into battle. It must recognize, also, that there are women who play seductress for their own narrow ends. But, when mean motives are stripped away, there are genuine ethical insights to be found. Uncovering them requires a detailed phenomenological analysis that must be guided by such questions as the following: What does the woman dread (beyond the loss of her man, his injury, her loneliness)? What tempts the man to defect (beyond the present sexual temptation)? What presses the woman to let him go? What drives him to leave? An exploration of these questions might reveal a deeply shared set of basic intuitions: that to be together sharing a life and building a family and community is better than to be alone or with valued others who are pledged to destruction; that a man who kills may never be quite like one who has not killed; that killing one who does not wish to die is somehow deeply wrong no matter who does it or in what cause; that human beings often fear the condemnation of their peers even more than death and loss; that separation induces the risk of lost love; that one's courage may fail and that one is not sure what courage is; that neglect of relation is itself a great evil (something we all once knew in our early fears of abandonment); that all people in a situation like ours—even those we are about to engage in combat—feel these things. All of these intuitions can be incorporated into a powerful ethical position that supports woman's way of being in the world as rational rather than weak or self-serving.

It is important to understand that it is not the purpose of such an analysis to claim or to demonstrate the moral superiority of women. No such claim is necessary. The aim is to pay attention to a perspective on ethical life that is available to us through women's experience and that may help all of us lead better lives. Daniel Maguire puts the matter well when he says, "Because the experience of women has given them certain advantages in their moral perceptivity, their exclusion from most centers of power in most civilizations has impoverished the species" (1982, pp. 59-60). I must add, however, that it is not just the exclusion of women that impoverishes the species; it is also the deprivation of experience in men. Because women's work, attitudes, and ways of thinking have been despised, men have avoided the sort of experience common to women. Therefore, the suggested analysis must probe *women's* experience for intuitions that may, with some modification, be shared by both men and women.

As the basic intuitions are uncovered, the value ascribed to them can be traced to tribal experience, as the Jungians have held. In contrast to the Jungians, however, we need not trace these differences beyond experience to essential differences in nature. This leaves open the possibility of both reconciliation and transcendence, while recognizing the difficulty of the enterprise. Men and women may be reconciled in appreciation of their differing experience and commitments; but they may also transcend the differences by a heroic effort to uncover what lies shared beneath the surface conflicts. What is it that man values in war? If it is power (macho-masculinity, tyranny), then we must reject it and call it evil, because it induces pain, separation, and helplessness. If it is faithfulness, adventure, challenge, and courage, then men and women may ask: How else can these aims and virtues be encouraged and indulged?

This begins to sound like a search for what William James called "the moral equivalent of war: something heroic that will speak to men as universally as war does, and yet will be as compatible with their spiritual selves as war has proved itself to be incompatible" (1958/1970, p. 284).[1] But the sense of James's statement suggests that he sought the motivational, not the moral, equivalent of war. His choice of words is, however, entirely consonant with the warrior mode and underscores my claim that the experience of men and women has been fundamentally different. Although he recognizes the incompatibility of war with a spiritual self, he still says, "Yet the fact remains that war is a school of strenuous life and heroism; and, being in the line of aboriginal instinct, is the only school that as yet is universally available" (p. 284). Women, looking at their own universe, might point to motherhood (also in line with aboriginal experience) as a school universally accessible and one that teaches very different lessons—lessons of tenderness, empowerment, and constancy (Gilligan 1982; Noddings 1984; Ruddick 1980). But James does not see this alternative. Indeed, he pursues the paradox of war's horror and glory by commenting, "But when we gravely ask ourselves whether this wholesale organization of irrationality and crime be our only bulwark against effeminacy, we stand aghast at the thought, and think more kindly of ascetic religion" (p. 284). Having the softer qualities of a woman is something against which men need a bulwark; it is not considered an alternative mode that has its own contribution to make to universal heroism. Indeed, a turn to ascetic religion as suggested by James reveals yet another familiar litany of "goods" that are accompanied by outcomes often regarded as evil by women: isolation and neglect of interpersonal relations, distrust and even abuse of the body and its desires, passionate attachment to abstraction and ritual instead of concrete others, a rejection of personal love in favor of universal love. James fears some of these, too, and is not entirely approving in his analysis of asceticism, but he fears "effeminacy" even more.

The longstanding fear of being like a woman or being captured by a woman has led men—even bright, open-minded men like James—to suppose that male experience must somehow be defined in opposition to female experience. James, who declared himself a pacifist and clearly deplored the horrors of war, was unable to let go of the male notions of "hardihood," "manliness," "striving," and the like. He found it necessary to cast about for experiential domains and activities that would provide a suitable arena for masculine prowess. I am not suggesting that virtues and traits honored by men be simply discarded; rather I am suggesting that they be analyzed anew from the perspective of women so that both women and men can be relieved of the burden of stereotypical expectations and of the violence and oppression that accompany them.

To articulate a feminine morality requires analysis of several kinds: first, the analysis of relational phenomena such as caring (Noddings 1984) and response (Gilligan 1982); second, the analysis of situations that have been used in the past to explicate male consciousness; third, the analysis of situations, tasks, and relations that are central to female experience; and fourth, the analysis of connections among the first three. What are the connections, if any, among the cultural and biological experience of women and (1) relational phenomena such as caring, response, and tenderness and (2) the traits, behaviors, and linguistic expressions that appear in situations already analyzed from the male perspective?

Such a program of analysis may well press a dialectic between male and female views of morality, and the outcome of a vigorous dialectic should be fuller and clearer vision of what it means to be a good person. It may also provide us with material to build the much needed morality of evil that was mentioned earlier. It is clear that, at the present time, most men would not regard themselves as fully human persons if they adopted a "feminine" moral attitude and, just as clearly, most women would not regard themselves as *good* if they employed the male mode exclusively.

LEARNING THE MANLY AND WOMANLY ARTS

Because the universal has been described by males, and culture has been created or at least interpreted by men, schools are pervaded by male language and structures. Although the manly arts of the warrior are no longer extensively and explicitly taught, they are embedded in literature and political history, in sports, in a controlling view of science, in academic contests, in the hierarchical structure of school districts, and in competition for grades. It is not just the presence of football teams and ROTC on campus that mark male dominance: rather, the standard curriculum itself may be characterized as a masculine project (Grumet 1981).

I am not going to argue it is wrong for boys (or girls) to learn the manly arts, but I do think it is wrong for them to be uncritically initiated into the warrior mode. Stories like the *Iliad* and *Odyssey* have been used for centuries to introduce young men to the virtues of the warrior model (Foster 1985) and young women to the model of the faithful wife. These stories need not be abandoned, but they should be examined critically; their characters and plots should not be allowed to stand as uncriticized exemplars of virtue. Further, young people should be encouraged to consider whether the tragic events in these stories are evil tricks of fate or whether they result from the warrior model itself—something evil embedded in it that ensures a continuous cycle of tragedy. Such critical examination is vitally important at the present time, because the differential effects of these stories on boys and girls may be fading. More and more, girls want access to the public world, and they may quite understandably emulate virtues that are presented to them as *human* virtues, even if those virtues are incompatible with the spiritual attitudes they have inherited from the maternal model.

Many people today, even many feminists, espouse an equity model. They assume that the cure for women's oppression is free and equitable access to the public world. They forget, however, that the public world has been defined and built by men. The standards and practices have been established by males and, thus, it is a male model women must adopt in availing themselves of free access. It is as though men were to say: "Here, now, we know that we have been unfair; we will now share our power and work with you; all you have to do is show that you're up to it." It is an unintentionally arrogant model that presupposes women want to be like men and just need the chance to grow in that direction. While I would not argue against equity, I would advise against a blind striving for equity without transformation; that is, I would argue against accepting equity in a model that promotes—and even glorifies—domination and oppression. The fundamental assumption here is that to be human is to be male.

An alternative is to analyze the structures and practices of our society from the perspective of women's experience and to begin the complex process of constructing a genuinely universal interpretation of culture. This is an extraordinarily difficult task, and only a few thinkers are working seriously at it. Jane Roland Martin (1984, 1985), for example, has suggested that we need to rethink our conception of the educated person, and our new ideal should be guided by a consideration of both "productive" and "reproductive" functions. She introduces these terms in a discussion of Plato's *Republic:*

A fascinating feature of the experiment in thought in which Socrates and his friends construct the Just State is that the reproductive processes of society are all but ignored. Socrates knows that in addition to cobblers, shipbuilders, and cowherds a state needs to have children born and reared, houses cared for, the sick and elderly tended, and everyone fed. Yet he mentions . . . occupations traditionally performed by females—only in passing (1985, p. 14).

I agree wholeheartedly with Martin's call for a new conception of the educated person, but I find her use of "productive" and "reproductive" problematic. The terms are usually found in Marxist settings and, thus, point to the economic status of the two sets of tasks; this emphasis does not serve Martin's purposes well. We cannot be sure, for example, whether child rearing in Martin's conceptual scheme moves from the reproductive to the productive when it becomes paid work, nor does that move matter to Martin in the way it would to a Marxist. We might infer from the body of Martin's work that it is not so much the tasks themselves that demarcate the productive and reproductive but a set of attitudes brought to the work; she herself identifies "caring, compassion, and connection" (p. 197). But if this is so, it underscores the need for a phenomenology of female experience, because these attitudes—this way of being in the world—have grown out of a relation to the tasks known as "women's work." As Martin points out, simply to say, for example, that we will now attend to the three Cs in school without studying and somehow including the activities that give rise to them is to fall into a peculiarly traditional abstractionism.

Martin recognizes that we cannot solve the curricular problem by adding courses such as "Compassion 101a," and she is also wary of "replicating within the curriculum the split between the productive and reproductive processes of society" (1985, p. 197). She would, therefore, oppose relegating the three Cs to courses like home economics. In this she is clearly right, but it may not be enough to attempt what she suggests in *Reclaiming A Conversation* as an alternative, namely "incorporating Sophie's and Sarah's [female] virtues into our science, math, history, literature, and auto mechanics courses, even as we emphasize theoretical knowledge and the development of reason in the teaching of nutrition or family living" (1985, p. 198).

The difficulty with this program is that it leaves the standard model very nearly intact; subject matter drawn from the traditional disciplines still reigns supreme. Martin recognizes this and has argued elsewhere for a dramatic change in subjects to be included in the curriculum (1970, 1977, 1982). If we truly want a universally representative culture and education, we need to revise both the curriculum as a whole *and* internal elements of the curriculum. The new subjects of the curriculum must, further, stand on an equal footing with geometry and physics; they must not be accorded second-class citizenship because they are developed from and reflect women's experience.

An example will illustrate the kind of change I see as necessary. Suppose we were to introduce a new subject called "People: Their Growth, Customs, and Relationships." This would not be a one semester course in anthropology, or social history, or psychology, or biology. Nor would it be interdisciplinary in the narrow sense of drawing directly and only upon these established disciplines. It would be an on-going subject with its own integrity—one taught across the years as math and English now are, and it would have a practice component. At the high school level, freshmen might study the young child and work directly as helpers in preschools and kindergartens. The course of study would include a history of childhood, classic works of art pertaining to childhood, children's poetry and literature (what a wonderful opportunity to revisit loved stories from a "higher" standpoint), the biology and developmental psychology of childhood, and some cross-cultural sociology of childhood.

Sophomores might study old age and do their practice in nursing homes and adult communities. A study of political action might be introduced: Should the elderly have special rights? How will the social security system be maintained? What happens when a society focuses on its elderly instead of its young?

Juniors might study systems of religion and morality. This would provide an opportunity for young people to learn not only about other religions but, perhaps more importantly, about the political agendas that have accompanied the development of their own religious systems. Study would include the great Judeo-Christian myths, their pagan predecessors, and their roles in the oppression and liberation of women. Practice in this course might be chosen from a variety of possibilities ranging from work with a particular religious institution to work or study within a secular group interested in the influence and role of religion. In this area of curriculum reform, cries about the separation of church and state are sure to be heard (at least in the United States). The reaction should be neither defiance nor capitulation. Rather, both those who recognize the positive contributions of religion to our culture and those who are convinced that religious institutions have conspired to support the warrior model should gently and persistently press the case. A tremendous mystique has grown up around this mythical "separation," and it is time to engage in demystification.

In their last year of high school, students might study interpersonal relations including sex, marriage, alternative life-styles, parenting, and friendship. Such courses already exist, of course, but not in the rich critical and practical patterns suggested here. All of these topics (and those of previous years as well) might be analyzed by examining the two great cultural models, warrior and mother.

This outline is, of course, a mere suggestion, and I am certainly not recommending that these topics—should they actually be selected—must be treated in this order. My main point is that subject matter can be defined and organized in a variety of ways. In particular, it can be organized around the topics that have been central to female experience. In a radical revision of education, the subjects themselves would be reconsidered and renamed in an attempt to achieve a vision of the humanities and sciences that would be more nearly universal. (I have been using the word *universal* in a descriptive, not prescriptive, sense; that is, I seek a cumulative description of moral life that includes voices long unheard in traditional attempts to build a universal prescriptive morality.)

I have argued that a new balance in education must draw as richly from female experience (in particular, the maternal model) as from male (the warrior model) and that this new balance requires a radical change in our conception of curriculum and subjects. In the meantime, the traditional subjects themselves must be reconsidered if children are to learn both the womanly and manly arts, and their learning must include both critical and appreciative analysis as well as appropriate practical experience in living out these models.

Clearly, an emphasis on female experience implies significant changes in school structure and pedagogy as well as curriculum, but I will concentrate here on curriculum. Two areas of the contemporary curriculum that might profit greatly from changes of content are English and social studies. I am not advocating the equity model which, in its most simplistic form, would merely urge upon us an inclusion of women in standard public roles. In English, not only must women writers be sought out but women's themes must be treated. Very few of our students are asked to read Pearl Buck's *The Exile* (1939), for example, even though both this book (a biography of her mother) and *Fighting Angel* (1964), a biography of her father, were named in her Nobel award. *The Exile* is a magnificent story of the suffering and constancy of a Victorian mother forever in conflict between her devotion to particular, bodily human beings and the abstract God she was called upon to worship. It portrays the agony induced by a society and church that regard care and compassion for bodies as morally inferior to care and concern for souls. At bottom, it illustrates the clash between mother (the exile) and warrior (fighting angel) and demonstrates, too, that both virtues and vices, strengths and weaknesses are found in each model.

In social studies, a complete reconstruction is necessary. Students need to learn how to be good neighbors as well as informed voters. They need the history of families, housing arrangements, food production, child raising, volunteer work, social reform, and religion. They should learn about the heroism of women and men who have worked for reform in our treatment of the insane, aged, immigrants, slaves, prisoners, workers, children, and animals. Furthermore, this material, so often buried in a few dull paragraphs, should be presented with drama and excitement, biography, and film.

The work to be done is enormous. Yet I agree with Jane Martin when she says that few tasks in education are as important or exciting (1985 p. 198). Martin also says that we should "not delude ourselves that education can be created anew" (1985, p. 198). This is certainly true of education seen as schooling. In our theoretical work, however, we *should* create education anew. The vision thus created can be used to guide the actual changes that we find feasible. Without such a vision, we grope blindly toward an unarticulated future. In achieving a fully human view of what it is to be a good person and in translating that view into an educational program, there is a need for a dialectic between male and female and also for one between the theoretical-ideal and the practical.

UNDERSTANDING AND CONTROLLING EVIL

Male and female conceptions of good and evil differ. In part, they differ because of the stereotypical expectations that have influenced all of us. A more interesting facet of the difference, however, appears when we see clearly how often and how dramatically men have defined themselves in op-position to all that is feminine. It is not just that women and men have been thought to be different but that maleness has been more often associated with the morally good and that evil has been defined in terms of disobe-dience of the patriarch. The analysis of women's experience with respect to evil may be even more important than the reevaluation of female virtues and traditional goodness. Again, it is vital to understand that this impor-tance is not rooted in a claim for women's perfection. As Maguire points out, "Our sisters are not without sin" (1982 p. 62). Rather, one great con-tribution of women's perspective arises from the very fact that women have been subordinated and forced to think of their own shortcomings. In Maguire's words, "[W]omen enjoy the wisdom that accrues to the alienated" (1982 p. 61). I'm not sure "alienated" is the right word; "powerless" might be better. But his meaning is clear: The experience of subordination can produce wisdom as well as the attitude Nietzsche calls a slave mentality. This is not, of course, an argument for the continuation of women's subordination. Rather, it is an argument for reflection on this ex-perience so that the wisdom accrued will not be lost as subordination is overcome.

Now that women are experiencing raised consciousness with respect to their long years of subordination, they are quite naturally interested in the political dimensions of programs and institutions, for example, the church, to which they have in the past given their uncritical devotion. As the religious heritage is examined, it becomes clear that dogma, doctrine, and custom have not grown solely out of spiritual concerns nor have they served only spiritual purposes. The story of Eve, for example, has been used to justify men's subordination of women and, in particular, to justify their close control over women's sexuality (Phillips 1984). Further, it now seems likely that parts of the Adam and Eve myth were designed to discredit and overthrow earlier female religions (Stone 1976; Sanford 1981). Looking at these stories with newly opened eyes, women are becoming keenly aware of the reasons and conditions under which evil has been defined as disobe-dience of the patriarch. This should be the right time, then, to undertake a phenomenology of evil from a female perspective.

What advantages might be found in using women's experience as a framework for the analysis of evil? First, women are in a peculiarly advan-tageous position to examine evil, because they have been treated as the "other" upon whom many evils have been projected (de Beauvoir 1952; Harding 1976). Second, because they have been relatively powerless to return the projection in the way that, say, two warring nations project evil on each other, they have learned to accept evil in themselves. Much of this is, of course, unwarranted, and I am not suggesting that the long associa-tion of women, materiality, and evil should be continued. It is neither the process of projection nor the projected content of evil that should be accepted but, rather, the healthy process of striving to bring unconscious evil into consciousness rather than repressing and projecting it.

In this area, the work of Jung and his followers should prove very useful, for their analysis clearly reveals the danger in failing to recognize and understand the evil in ourselves. Jung (1969) even suggests that the Christian view of God as all-good needs to be revised to incorporate an evil side of the deity. In his recommendations for the conscious recognition of evil in both deity and human, Jung is not arguing for uncritical acceptance of evil or for a new power in performing evil deeds. Rather, he is arguing that wholeness requires a controlled acceptance and understanding of the evil in ourselves and that this acceptance gives us some protection from actually committing evil.

Although there is wisdom in the Jungian teaching, there is also cause for feminist concern. When Jung discusses what is missing in the Christian view of God—what needs to be added to make a "whole" picture of God—he sometimes identifies the missing element as the evil side and sometimes identifies it as the feminine! Clearly, an uncritical reading of Jung could be used to sustain the traditional equation of women and evil. A more careful reading suggests that incorporation of the feminine may be a necessary prelude to the acceptance of evil in oneself and an end to projection of evil onto an "other." When the other is an integral part of oneself, what-is-there must be faced, controlled, improved, and treated with some respect. The experience of women in living as other should, clearly, be a valuable resource in our study of wholeness and its relation to evil.

What does all this suggest for education? First, of course, it suggests the need to add feminine interpretations of the history of religion to our curriculum. It is critically important that young women and men learn what the Judeo-Christian tradition has done for them and to them. Any education that purports to be liberal is a fraud without this body of knowledge.

Second, it suggests the need for more attention to self-knowledge in the curriculum. This recommendation—in the context of good and evil—is compatible with similar suggestions now being made by scholars interested in meta-cognition. They, too, recommend that students learn more about their own thought processes and the affects that enhance or impede them. A feminine approach to moral education would include what we learn from a morality of evil. Students would learn not only about the long history of attempts to project evil onto others but also would be helped to explore and bring to consciousness their own shadow sides. (The shadow, it should be noted, is not always evil; it contains subordinated elements that are good as well.) Self-knowledge is as important to the moral side of education as it is to the intellectual side.

Finally, programs in critical thinking—especially those that focus on social studies—should include studies that help students to understand how people are manipulated by leaders and governments into projecting evil onto other human beings called enemies. Most social studies programs today include some discussion of the injustices committed by our own government but very few explore directly and systematically the ways in which people are made into enemies. High school students learn, for example, that the Germans and Japanese were our enemies in World War II and that they are now among our allies, but they do not hear war songs like "We've got to slap the dirty little Jap" nor do they hear General MacArthur say as he wades ashore stepping over dead Japanese bodies, "That's the way I like to see them." Students thoroughly educated about their national shadow might be less likely to condemn Russians as citizens of an "evil empire" or to assume that Libyans deserve to be bombed because they follow an evil leader. The study of good and evil from a feminine perspective is essential to both personal and national wholeness.

SUMMARY

I have made two kinds of suggestions in this chapter. On a theoretical level, I have suggested the need for phenomenologies of good and evil from the perspective of feminine experience.

On the level of practice, I have suggested that an education aimed at producing good people must include feminine perspectives on good and evil. Both girls and boys need to know about the traditional association of women with evil and how religious myths have been used to maintain the subordination of women. All students need, also, to study and practice the womanly arts of caring for children, the sick, elderly, and needy; they need to learn how to initiate and maintain stable and gratifying relationships and how to run households in a way that nourishes bodies, minds, and spirits. They need to study the warrior model both critically and appreciatively so that its enduring virtues can be transposed to a less violent mode of living and interacting with others. Finally, they need to gain greater self-knowledge through studies that help them to accept their personal and group shadow sides. Until this material is incorporated in our school curriculum, we can hardly claim honestly that our aim is to produce good people.

NOTE

1. James wrote an essay entitled "The Moral Equivalent of War" that was widely circulated in 1910 (see James, 1958/1970). The quotations here are from James's Gifford Lectures (1901) that later appeared as *The Varieties of Religious Experience*.

REFERENCES

Augustine. *On free will*, III, *ix*, 26.
Barrett, W. (1962). *Irrational man*. Garden City, NY: Doubleday Anchor.

De Beauvoir, S. (1952). *The second sex*. Trans. and ed. H. M. Parshley. New York: Random House.

Bernard, J. (1975). *The future of motherhood*. New York and Baltimore: Penguin Books.

Black, N. (1983). Virginia Woolf: The life and happiness. In *Feminist theories*, ed. D. Spencer. New York: Pantheon Books.

Buck, P. (1939). *The exile*. New York: Triangle Books.

_____ . (1964). *Fighting angel*. New York: Pocket Books.

Chodorow, N. (1978). *The reproduction of mothering: Psychoanalysis and the sociology of gender*. Berkeley: University of California Press.

Daly, M. (1974). *Beyond God the Father*. Boston: Beacon Press.

_____ . (1984). *Pure lust*. Boston: Beacon Press.

Dinnerstein, D. (1976). *The mermaid and the minotaur: Sexual arrangements and human malaise*. New York: Harper Colophon.

Erikson, E. (1969). *Gandhi's truth*. New York: W. W. Norton.

Foster, B. G. (1985). Facing the gods: Archetypal images of father and son in *The Odyssey*. *Independent School* 44(3):Symposium 8-20.

Von Franz, M. (1983). *Shadow and evil in fairy tales*. Dallas: Spring.

Gilligan, C. (1982). *In a different voice*. Cambridge: Harvard University Press.

Grumet, M. (1981). Conception, contradiction and curriculum. *Journal of Curriculum Theorizing* 3(1):287-298.

Harding, M. E. (1976). *Woman's mysteries*. New York: Harper Colophon.

James, W. (1958/1970). The moral equivalent of war. In *War and Morality*, ed. R. A. Wasserstrom. Belmont, CA: Wadsworth.

_____ . (1958). *The varieties of religious experience*. New York: Mentor.

Jung, C. G. (1969). Answer to Job. In *Psychology and religion*, Vol. 2 of the Collected Works. Princeton: Princeton/Bollinger.

Maguire, D. C. (1982). The feminization of God and ethics. *Christianity and crisis*, March 15, 59-67.

Martin, J. R. (1985). *Reclaiming a conversation*. New Haven and London: Yale University Press.

_____ . (1984). Bringing women into educational thought. *Educational Theory* 34(4):341-354.

_____ . (1982). Two dogmas of curriculum. *Synthese* 5(1):5-20.

_____ . (1977). The anatomy of subjects. *Educational Theory* 27(2):86-95.

_____ . (1970). The disciplines and the curriculum. In *Readings in the philosophy of education: A study of curriculum*, ed. J. R. Martin. Boston: Allyn & Bacon.

Neumann, E. (1955). *The great mother*. Princeton: Princeton University Press.

Nietzsche, F. (1886/1973). *Beyond good and evil*. London: Penguin.

Noddings, N. (1984). *Caring: A feminine approach to ethics and moral education*. Berkeley: University of California Press.

Phillips, J. A. (1984). *Eve: The history of an idea*. New York: Harper & Row.

Ricoeur, P. (1969). *The symbolism of evil*. Boston: Beacon Press.

Ruddick, S. (1980). Maternal thinking, *Feminist Studies* 6(2):342-367.

_____ . (1984). Preservative love and military destruction: Some reflections on mothering and peace. In *Mothering: Essays in feminist theory*, ed. J. Trebilcot. Totowa, NJ: Rowman and Allanheld.

Ruether, R. R. (1983). *Sexism and God-talk*. Boston: Beacon Press.
Sanford, J. A. (1981). *Evil*: *The shadow side of reality*. New York: Crossroad.
Stone, M. (1976). *When God was a woman*. San Diego, New York, London: Harvest/Harcourt Brace Jovanovich.

Selected Bibliography

Andolsen, B. H. (1986). *Daughters of Jefferson, daughters of bootblacks*: *Racism and American feminism*. Macon, GA: Mercer University Press.

Andolsen, B. H., Gudorf, C. E., and Pellauer, M. D. (1985). *Women's consciousness, women's conscience*. Minneapolis, MN: Winston Press.

Auerbach, J., Blum, L., Smith, V., and Williams, C. (1985). Commentary on Gilligan's *In a Different Voice*. *Feminist Studies* 11:149-161.

Baier, A. (1985). What do women want in moral theory? *Nous* 1:53-63.

_____ . (1986). Trust and antitrust. *Ethics* 96:231-260.

Baumrind, D. (1986). Sex differences in moral reasoning: Response to Walker's (1984) conclusion that there are none. *Child Development* 57:511-521.

Belenky, M., Clinchy, B., Goldberger, N., and Tarule, J. (1986). *Women's ways of knowing*. New York:Basic Books.

Bell-Scott, P., and Guy-Sheftall, B., eds. (1984). Mothers and daughters. [Special Issue]. *Sage: A Journal of Black Women* 1 (2).

Benhabib, S. (1986). The generalized and the concrete other: The Kohlberg-Gilligan controversy and feminist theory. *Praxis International* 5(4):402-424.

Blum, L. (1980). *Friendship, altruism, and morality*. London: Routledge and Kegan.

Brabeck, M., ed. (1987). Feminist perspectives on moral education and development. [Special Issue]. *Journal of Moral Education* 16 (3).

_____ . (1983). Moral judgment: Theory and research on differences between males and females. *Developmental Review* 3(3):274-291.

Brown, L., Argyris, D., Attanucci, J., Bardige, B., Gilligan, C., Johnston, K., Miller, B., Osborne, D., Ward, J., Wiggins, G., and Wilcox, D. (1988). *A guide to reading narratives of conflict and choice for self and moral voice*. Center for the Study of Gender, Education and Human Development, Harvard University.

Brown, L. M., Tappan, M. B., Gilligan, C., Miller, B. A., and Argyris, D. E. (In press). Reading for self and moral voice: A method for interpreting narratives of real-life moral conflict and choice. In *Interpretive investigations: Contributions to psychological research*, ed. M. Packer and R. Addison. Binghamton: SUNY Press.

Cancian, F. (1987). *Love in America: Gender and self-development*. Cambridge: Cambridge University Press.

Carlson, M. (1988). *Feminismo!: The woman's movement in Argentina from its beginnings to Eva Perón*. Chicago: Academy Chicago Publishers.

Chodorow, N. (1978). *The reproduction of mothering: Psychoanalysis and the sociology of gender*. Berkeley, CA: University of California Press.

Daly, M. (1974). *Beyond God the Father*. Boston: Beacon Press.

———. (1984). *Pure lust*. Boston: Beacon Press.

Davis, A. Y. (1981). *Women, race, and class*. New York: Random House.

Dinnerstein, D. (1976). *The mermaid and the minotaur: Sexual arrangements and human malaise*. New York: Harper Colophon.

Eisenberg, N. (1986). *Altruistic emotion, cognition and behavior*. Hillsdale, NJ: Lawrence Erlbaum Associates.

Eisenberg, N. and Strayer, J., eds. (1987). *Empathy and its development*. Cambridge: Cambridge University Press.

Eisenstein, H. (1983). *Contemporary feminist thought*. Boston: G. K. Hall & Co.

Flanagan, O. (1982). Virtue, sex and gender: Some philosophical reflections on the moral psychology debate. *Ethics* 92:501.

Flanagan, O., and Jackson, K. (1987). Justice, care and gender: The Kohlberg-Gilligan debate revisited. *Ethics* 97:622-637.

Ford, M. R., and Lowery, C. R. (1986). Gender differences in moral reasoning: A comparison of the use of justice and care orientations. *Journal of Personality and Social Psychology* 50:777-783.

French, M. (1985). *Beyond power: On women, men, and morals*. New York: Ballentine Books.

Friedman, M. (1985). *Care and context in moral reasoning*. MOSAIC monograph no. 1. Bath, England: University of Bath Press.

Gilligan, C. (1982). *In a different voice: Psychological theory and women's development*. Cambridge, MA: Harvard University Press.

———. (1986). Exit-voice/dilemmas in adolescent development. In *Development, democracy, and the art of trespassing*, ed. A. Foley, M. McPherson, and G. O'Donnell. Indiana: University of Notre Dame Press.

Gilligan, C. and Belenky, M. (1980). A naturalistic study of abortion decisions. In *New Directions for Child Development*, ed. R. Selman and R. Yando. San Francisco: Josey-Bass.

Gilligan, C., Langdale, C., Lyons, N., and Murphy, J. M. (1982). *The contribution of women's thought to developmental theory*. Final Report to the National Institute of Education. Cambridge, MA: Harvard University.

Gilligan, C., and Lyons, N. (1985). *Listening to voices we have not heard*. Report to the New York State Department of Education on the Emma Willard Study. Cambridge, MA: Harvard University.

Gilligan, C., and Wiggins, G. (1987). The origins of morality in early childhood relationships. In *The emergence of morality in young children*, ed. J. Kagan and S. Lamb. Chicago: University of Chicago Press.

Haan, N., Bellah, R. N., Rabinow, P., and Sullivan, W. M., eds. (1983). *Social science as moral inquiry*. New York: Columbia University Press.

Hayles, N. K. (1986). Anger in different voices: Carol Gilligan and *The Mill on the Floss*. *Signs: Journal of Women in Culture and Society* 12:23-39.

Hsu, F. L. K. (1983). *Rugged individualism reconsidered: Essays in psychological anthropology*. Knoxville, TN: The University of Tennessee Press.

Hull, G. T., Scott, P. B., and Smith, B. eds. (1982). *All the women are white, all the blacks are men, but some of us are brave*. Old Westbury, NY: Feminist Press.

Hyde, J. S., and Linn, M. C., eds. (1986). *The psychology of gender: Advances through meta-analysis*. Baltimore: Johns Hopkins University Press.

Jones, J. (1986). *Labor of love, labor of sorrow: Black women, work, and the family from slavery to the present*. New York: Vintage Books.

Jordan, J. V. (1984). *Empathy and self boundaries*. (Working Papers in Progress, No. 85-05.) Wellesley, MA: Wellesley College, The Stone Center.

Joseph, G., and Lewis, J., eds. (1981). *Common differences: Conflicts in black and white feminist perspectives*. Garden City, NY: Anchor Press/Doubleday.

Kaplan, A. G. (1984). *The "self-in-relation": Implications for depression in women*. (Working Papers in Progress, No. 84-03.) Wellesley, MA: Wellesley College, The Stone Center.

Kerber, L. K., Greeno, C. G., Maccoby, E. E., Luria, Z., Stack, C. B., and Gilligan, C. (1986). On *In a Different Voice*: An interdisciplinary forum. *Signs: Journal of Women in Culture and Society* 11(2):304-333.

Kittay, E. F., and Meyers, D. T., eds. (1987). *Women and moral theory*. Totowa, NJ: Rowman & Littlefield.

Kohlberg, L. (1984). *The psychology of moral development*. San Francisco: Harper and Row.

Kohlberg, L., Levine, C., and Hewer, A. (1983). *Moral stages: A current formulation and a response to critics*. Basel: S. Karger.

Lindsey, B., ed. (1978). *Comparative perspectives of third world women: The impact of race, sex, and class*. New York: Praeger Publishers.

Lowe, M., and Hubbard, R., eds. (1983). *Woman's nature: Rationalizations of inequality*. New York: Pergamon Press.

Lykes, M. B. (1985). Gender and individualistic vs. collectivist bases for notions about the self. *Journal of Personality* 53(2):357-383.

Lyons, N. (1981). *Manual for coding responses to the question: How would you describe yourself to yourself?* Unpublished manuscript, Harvard University.

Lyons, N. (1983). Two perspectives: On self, relationships, and morality. *Harvard Educational Review* 53:125-145.

Martin, J. R. (1984). Bringing women into educational thought. *Educational Theory* 34:341-354.

_____ . ed. (1970). *Readings in the philosophy of education*. Boston: Allyn & Bacon.

_____ . (1985). *Reclaiming a conversation: The ideal of the educated woman*. New Haven: Yale Univesity Press.

Mayeroff, P. M. (1971). *On caring*. New York: Harper & Row.

Miller, J. B. (1984). *The development of women's sense of self*. (Working Papers in Progress, No. 84-01.) Wellesley, MA: Wellesley College, The Stone Center.

———. (1976). *Toward a new psychology of women*. Boston: Beacon Press.

Nails, D., O'Loughlin, M. A., and Walker, J. C., eds. (1983). Women and morality. [Special Issue]. *Social Research* 50(3).

Nicholson, L. (1983). Women, morality and history. *Social Research* 50(3):514-536.

Noddings, N. (1984). *Caring: A feminine approach to ethics and moral education*. Berkeley, CA: University of California Press.

Nunner-Winkler, G. (1984). Two moralities? A critical discussion of an ethics of care and responsibility versus an ethics of rights and justice. In *Morality, moral behavior and moral development*, ed. W. M. Kurtines and J. L. Gewirtz. New York: Wiley.

Pratt, M. W., Golding, G., and Hunter, W. J. (1984). Does morality have a gender? Sex, sex role, and moral judgment relationships across the adult life span. *Merrill-Palmer Quarterly* 30:321-348.

Reiter, R. R., ed. (1975). *Toward an anthropology of women*. New York: Monthly Review Press.

Rose, L. R. (1980). *The black woman*. Beverly Hills, CA: Sage Publications.

Rothbart, M. K., Hanley, D., and Albert, M. (1986). Gender differences in moral reasoning. *Sex Roles* 15:645-653.

Ruddick, S. (1980). Maternal thinking. *Feminist Studies* 6(2):342-367.

———. (1985). Maternal work and the practice of peace. *Journal of Education* 167(3):97–111.

Shogan, D. (1988). *Care and moral motivation*. Toronto, Ontario: OISE Press.

Sichel, B. A. (1985). Women's moral development in search of philosophical assumptions. *Journal of Moral Education* 14(3):149-161.

Stewart, A. J., and Lykes, M. B., eds. (1985). *Gender and personality: Current perspectives on theory and research*. Durham, NC: Duke University Press.

Thoma, S. (1986). Estimating gender differences in the comprehension and preference of moral issues. *Developmental Review* 6:165-180.

Trebilcot, J., ed. (1984). *Mothering*. Totowa, NJ: Rowman and Allenheld.

Tronto, J. C. (1987). Beyond gender difference to a theory of care. *Signs: Journal of Women in Culture and Society* 12(4):644-663.

Waithe, M. E., ed. (1987). *A history of women philosophers*, Vol. 1. Dordrecht: Martinus Nijoff Publishers.

Walker, L. (1984). Sex differences in the development of moral reasoning: A critical review. *Child Development* 55:677-691.

———. (1989). A longitudinal study of moral reasoning. *Child Development* 60:157-166.

Walker, L. J. (1986). Sex differences in the development of moral reasoning: A rejoinder to Baumrind. *Child Development* 57:522-526.

Walker, L. J., deVries, B., and Trevethan, S. D. (1987). Moral stages and moral orientations in real life and hypothetical dilemmas. *Child Development* 58:842-858.

Index

63–82; sexism effects on women, 29–34; slave mentality, 218; slavery and black women, 51–53; socioeconomics of black women, 48–51; stereotypes between the sexes, 128–29; transaction of, 189–91; undifferentiated moral theory and, 3–15; values and, 78–80; womanly arts, 223–27; worthy caring relations and social context, 90–98

gender differences: caring self, 164–77; contextualism and, 76–78; "different voice" (Gilligan), 19–42; educating moral people, 216–30; empathy, 127–40; empathy and, 130–32; empathy and empirical findings, 133–36; ethical sensitivity among men and women in the profession, 144–60; expression of care, 197–214; expression of justice, 197–214; female perspective in moral education, 220–23; feminism as social policy, 201; feminism values clarification in education, 202–04; genderized traits, 189–91; good and evil differences, 227–30; just community approach, 72–76; just community educational program, 197–214; manly arts, 223–27; moral reasoning and, 64–72, 136–37; moral sensitivity as a theoretical construct, 151–52; moral theory and, 7; prosocial moral judgment empirical findings, 137–39; prosocial moral reasoning, 127–40; in reasoning ability, 13–14; roles in, 128; second gender undifferentiated view, 8; self-report data in, 135; sense of self, 165–69; slave mentality, 218; socialization of emotion, 129–30; socialization of empathy, 132–33; social morality and, 6; in Spanish philosophy, 12; subjugation and liberation and, 21–23; sympathetic caring and, 80–82; sympathy and empirical findings, 133–36; third version, 14–15;

transactions of gender, 189–91; values and, 78–80; womanly arts, 223–27

gender undifferentiated moral theory, 3–15; definition of, 4; in Greek philosophy, 6; second view evolution, 8; women philosophers and, 11–14. *See also* justice

Gibbs, J., 147
Gibbs, J. C., 137, 146, 152
Giddings, Paula, 52, 55
Gilkes, C. T., 47
Gilligan, Carol, 3–6, 15, 19–43, 51–52, 54, 63, 65, 67, 69, 85–90, 94–95, 99, 106–8, 122, 127, 129, 136–37, 145–46, 148, 164–70, 183, 194, 199, 222–23
Goldberger, N., 121–23
Golding, G., 148
good and evil: conflict over, 216–20
Goodlad, J. I., 185
Goodman, Ellen, 91–93
Gray, J. G., 184, 191
Greek philosophy, 5, 11; social morality and, 6
Grief des dames (Gournay), 12
Grief, E., 130
Grimshaw, Jean, 94–95
Grumet, M., 222
Gutman, H., 52
Guy-Sheftall, B., 169
Gwaltney, James Langston, 171

Haccoun, D. M., 128
Hand, M., 138
Hanley, D., 148
Harding, M. E., 217, 220, 228
Hart, H. L. A., 191
Hartmann, D. P., 145
Hartshorne, H., 202
Havighurst, J. R., 202, 302
Haviland, J. M., 130
Heloise, 11
Hemons, W. M., 47
Hersh, R. H., 183–84
Hewer, A., 147
Higgin, A., 147
Higginbotham, E., 56

Editor and Contributors

MARY BRABECK, Associate Professor, School of Education, Boston College, Chestnut Hill, Massachusetts

MURIEL J. BEBEAU, Associate Professor, School of Dentistry, University of Minnesota, Minneapolis, Minnesota

NANCY EISENBERG, Professor, Department of Psychology, Arizona State University, Tempe, Arizona

TOINETTE M. EUGENE, Provost, Colgate Rochester Divinity School, Crozer Theological Seminary, Rochester, New York

RICHARD FABES, Associate Professor, Department of Family Resources and Human Development, Arizona State University, Tempe, Arizona

ANN HIGGINS, Lecturer, Graduate School of Education, Harvard University, Cambridge, Massachusetts

BARBARA HOUSTON, Associate Professor, Department of Educational Policy Studies, University of Western Ontario, London, Ontario, Canada

M. BRINTON LYKES, Associate Professor, Department of Psychology, Rhode Island College, Providence, Rhode Island

NONA LYONS, Lecturer, Graduate School of Education, Harvard University, Cambridge, Massachusetts

JANE ROLAND MARTIN, Professor, Philosophy Department, University of Massachusetts, Harbor Campus, Boston, Massachusetts

NEL NODDINGS, Professor, School of Education, Stanford University, Stanford, California

BILL PUKA, Associate Professor, Rensselaer Polytechnic Institute, Troy, New York

CHARLENE HADDOCK SEIGFRIED, Associate Professor, Department of Philosophy, Purdue University, West Lafayette, Indiana

CINDY SHEA, Graduate Student, Department of Psychology, Arizona State University, Tempe, Arizona

MARY ELLEN WAITHE, Research Associate, Department of Health Ecology, School of Dentistry, University of Minnesota, Minneapolis, Minnesota